Understanding Pain

Understanding Pain

Exploring the Perception of Pain

Fernando Cervero

The MIT Press
Cambridge, Massachusetts
London, England

MIT Press books may be purchased at special quantity discounts for business or sales promotional use. For information, please email special_sales@mitpress.mit.edu or write to Special Sales Department, The MIT Press, 55 Hayward Street, Cambridge, MA 02142.

Set in Syntax and Times Roman by Toppan Best-set Premedia Limited. Printed and bound in the United States of America.

Library of Congress Cataloging-in-Publication Data

Cervero, Fernando.
Understanding pain : exploring the perception of pain / Fernando Cervero.
p. cm.
Includes index.
ISBN 978-0-262-01804-3 (hardcover : alk. paper)
1. Pain. 2. Pain perception. 3. Pain—Treatment. I. Title.
RB127.C43 2012
616'.0472—dc23
                                                    2012003899

10 9 8 7 6 5 4 3 2 1

for Pedro (Pete), Andrés (Andy), and Louisa (Luisi), with all my love
(and an apology)

in memoriam: Ainsley Iggo (1924–2012)

Pleasure and pain and that which causes them, good and evil, are the hinges on which our passions turn.
—John Locke, 1690

The answer, my friend, is blowin' in the wind / The answer is blowin' in the wind
—Bob Dylan, 1963

Contents

Preface

A three-year-old boy has just fallen off a swing in a playground. He has injured his knee, the skin is torn, and there is a little blood coming from the wound. He cries and cries, because it hurts a lot. His mother gives him a big hug, washes the wound, and applies a little antiseptic. She knows that it is nothing serious and that it will happen again anyway. And, predictably, she tells him "Big boys don't cry."

The boy will quickly learn that pain is an essential part of life. There will be more scrapes and grazes in playgrounds, falls from bicycles, perhaps even a broken bone. There will be visits to dentists, a surgical procedure, injections, and muscle aches. As he grows into adolescence, a girl will break his heart and a different form of pain, invisible but no less real, will also make him cry. Later in life he will suffer from arthritis, heart disease, and perhaps cancer. Physicians will tell him again and again that he must learn to live with his pain. By the end of his life, he will have endured a great deal of pain with dignity and resilience. He will know very well that pain is inevitable and that big boys don't cry.

Girls too learn very quickly that pain is an essential part of life. By age 12 or 13, they begin to experience a process of periodic pains that will remind them forever of their womanhood. For many there will also be the pain of childbirth and later in life, they will suffer from diseases (such as migraine, fibromyalgia, or irritable bowel syndrome) that are several times as prevalent in women as in men. And, although they may be allowed to have a little cry every now and then, they will also be told by their partners, their physicians, their midwives, and their mothers to pull themselves together and stop being hysterical.

In my professional environment—that is, among scientists who study pain mechanisms and physicians who treat patients—pain is often described as a multidimensional phenomenon, an expression that sounds boring and academic, but that conveys quite well the nature of this

complex feeling. Pain's influence on our lives is far greater than that of any other neurological process. Pain is our most powerful emotion, an essential learning tool, a major factor in our relationship with the world, and the source of much of our social behavior. Its many dimensions include physical responses, emotional reactions, rational thoughts, social influences, and spiritual feelings.

Consider, for example, the pain that we feel when we touch something hot. The sensation is very intense, and it triggers an immediate withdrawal from the hot object and a strong aversive emotion. These are useful and protective reactions, and we cannot do without them. People born without the ability to feel pain are continually injuring themselves and putting their lives at risk. This kind of pain is good for us. It is a protective component of our sensory repertoire, an alarm signal that warns of danger and keeps us out of harm. Yet if pain persists, if it becomes chronic, if an injury fails to heal quickly, or if pain appears without an apparent cause, this protective sensation becomes a nightmare, a curse, something that we want to get rid of by any means possible. The feeling of pain doesn't change; it remains unpleasant and emotionally negative, but its significance to our lives undergoes a dramatic switch from good and protective to awful and nasty. No other sensory process can change so radically from a defensive feeling to a curse.

Thus, not only is pain a complex biological process, sensory, emotional, and rational, but it is also a component of our lives that can be, at the same time, a helpful friend and our greatest foe. These remarkable properties generate two fundamental questions: How do we feel pain? What does pain mean to us?

The first question is purely mechanistic. From a biological point of view, and knowing that pain is a product of brain function, how is it that a sensory process meant as a warning and as a protective signal can degenerate into a dreadful feeling that destroys our lives? What happens in the brain so that a normal and useful component of our sensory equipment can be transformed into a source of intense suffering? To answer this question, we must explore the workings of the brain, our mechanisms for the detection of injury, and how the plasticity of these mechanisms forces them to switch from friend to foe. The study of pain, both normal and abnormal, is intrinsic to the scientific quest to understand the workings of the human brain.

The second question is more general and somewhat philosophical. How does pain influence our lives? Is it a test of our courage and resilience, or should we make every effort to eliminate it? Pain has been

regarded since the beginning of recorded history as a curse on mankind and a punishment for sin, and this has encouraged an attitude of inevitability, resignation, and acceptance. But as science moves forward and we learn more about how to influence the activity of our brain, including the perception of pain, we can also reduce or even eliminate pain from life. With epidural analgesia, giving birth is no longer painful. Surgical operations, even complex ones, don't generate intense pain if appropriate postoperative analgesia is available. Chronic diseases are not painful if analgesics are added to the treatments. And when we arrive at the end of our journey, we want a dignified and painless exit. Modern society demands a pain-free life and a pain-free end to life.

As our scientific knowledge increases, these two questions become interconnected. Advances in genetics have influenced current opinion on disease prevention and have radically affected how we view human reproduction. The ability to live a longer life has changed social attitudes about the age structure of a useful workforce but has also brought end-of-life questions to the forefront. And, as we know more about the mechanisms of pain, how to control pain, and how to keep pain from becoming chronic, the traditional view of pain as a test of character that must be accepted and endured is also crumbling. No more suffering in silence, no more painful agony.

Statistics tell us that about a third of the people in the world live with pain. In developing countries, pain is commonplace, a familiar ingredient of everyday life. Many hospitals and clinics lack sufficient resources to offer their patients adequate pain control, and people suffer through their diseases and die in agony. In developed countries, the prevalence of chronic pain increases with age; as the population gets older, the sum total of pain becomes progressively greater. And yet, because social attitudes toward pain are changing in both the developed and the developing worlds, the demand for more and better analgesia is also increasing. Greater scientific knowledge has triggered a change in social attitude that in turn has brought pain prevention and pain treatment to the forefront of our awareness. Indeed, several professional organizations around the world are campaigning for recognition of pain treatment as a fundamental human right.

So, what is pain and how does pain influence our life? Being very much aware that, as H. L. Mencken wrote, "there is always a well-known solution to every human problem: neat, plausible, and wrong," I want to examine the meaning of pain by asking questions rather than by providing definite answers. Pain is a brain function and therefore the focal point

of the inquiry is the scientific examination of what we know about the neural mechanisms of pain. And I must, from the start, make a disclaimer: I will not try to provide an encyclopedic description of all that is currently known about pain mechanisms. A great deal of excellent information about these mechanisms is published in scientific journals and books and, this being a fast-moving field, much of this information is changing rapidly.

This book is also the result of a life-long ambition. Ever since I began to study the mechanisms of pain, more than 35 years ago, I tried to bring some order, first in my own mind and then in the minds of my colleagues, to what I perceived as a research field often based on misunderstandings and confusions. I have always had a rather neurotic taste for order and tidiness, and the study of pain mechanisms has offered me an endless source of things to tidy up. Over the years, I wrote down, in notebooks and on scraps of paper, questions and thoughts on how injury is detected and processed by the brain, how some of these signals become pain perceptions, and what these feelings mean to us and to our society. The intention, or better the dream, was that perhaps one day I could collect these thoughts in a book. At last the opportunity came up, and here is the result. Writing this book has helped me to polish my own ideas and to discover new thoughts about a subject that has influenced my life for decades. If readers feel that the book has also helped them to think about what pain is and what it means to their lives, I will have succeeded.

Two individuals are directly responsible for making this project a reality. I was first approached and encouraged to write this book by Amanda Cushman. I am extremely grateful to her for suggesting a vehicle for this venture and for introducing me to Bob Prior, Executive Editor at the MIT Press, who further supported the project and provided considerable help and advice. Writing the book has taken much longer than I originally planned, and I am sure that Amanda and Bob are both familiar with this problem. Their support and editorial expertise have been essential to getting the job done.

Many of the ideas in this book are products of discussions and debates with numerous co-workers and colleagues. The list is very long, and I will take the risk of offending them all by not mentioning their individual names. The one exception is Jenny Laird, my most frequent co-author and co-worker and the person with whom I have talked the most about pain research, not only in the laboratory but also at home, for I have shared my life with her for the last 20 years. Our daughter Louisa has had to endure listening to us talking shop every evening over dinner;

when she was in elementary school, she told us one night that she was the only kid in her class who knew what TRPV1 receptors were, and this made us feel very guilty. Louisa was a strong driving force in the writing of this book, telling me almost every day to get on with it. The book is dedicated to her and to my two sons, Pedro and Andrés. They are my greatest source of pride, and living proof that pleasure and pain are inseparable components of our emotions. To them and to all the people who have helped me in this quest, my heartfelt thanks.

1 A Biological Enigma: The Meaning of Pain

Charles Sherrington, one of the greatest neuroscientists of all time, defined pain in a textbook on physiology published in 1900 as "the psychical adjunct of a protective reflex." We touch something hot and our brain triggers a reflex action that causes us to withdraw our hand from the object and thus protects us from injury. And to help us to learn and understand that touching something hot is dangerous, the brain produces an unpleasant sensation in parallel with the protective action: "the psychical adjunct of a protective reflex." It is hard to say more about pain with just seven words. It is also a beautiful use of the English language—a clear, concise, to-the-point definition.

Sherrington was a great scholar, a student of the nervous system whose interest on the human brain workings, and its output, went well beyond the details of purely mechanistic analyses. His thorough education and his knowledge of classical languages are evident in his writings. He wanted to understand the higher functions of the brain, such as memory, reasoning, and willpower, by studying the elementary neural networks that are the building blocks of the nervous system. He saw the brain as a complex building whose basic structure was the *reflex*, a simple chain of nerve cells. He thought that the progressive development of more complex reflexes and networks generates the properties that make the human brain unique and powerful. He proposed that every brain function is the result of a balance of excitation and inhibition of neural networks that he called *integration*, and that the building blocks of integrative action are the cellular structures that form the contacts between adjacent neurons. The Spanish histologist Santiago Ramón y Cajal had shown, at the end of the nineteenth century, that nerve cells don't fuse with one another but rather maintain a small gap between their contacts, through which messages flow in neural networks. Sherrington called these junctions *synapses*, a term derived from a Greek word meaning "to

fasten together." Sherrington's understanding of the brain as a progressively complex structure of elementary networks of nerve cells that
communicate with one another through their synaptic contacts remains
today as the fundamental interpretation of brain function. His legacy to
neuroscience is immense.

Sherrington's views on pain as a brain function are also highly significant. The most important element of his definition is the separation of
perception from processing. We can understand the protective-reflex
component of the definition, and we can use this approach to identify
the networks of nerve cells that mediate the reflexive withdrawal of a
body part that saves it from injury. But what is the nature of this psychical
adjunct? Can we explain what pain is, or how pain feels, to someone who
hasn't had a similar pain experience? Other students of pain mechanisms
have acknowledged their frustration when trying to define pain or have
refused to come up with a definition. In a brilliant book on pain mechanisms published in 1942, the Welsh neurologist Thomas Lewis wrote:
"Reflection tells me that I am so far from being able satisfactorily to
define pain, of which I here write, that the attempt could serve no useful
purpose", and added: "pain is known to us by experience and described
by illustration." James MacKenzie, a Scottish surgeon who in 1909 published a book on the mechanistic interpretation of pain symptoms, also
confessed his frustration with definitions of pain: "Pain is a disagreeable
sensation which everyone has experienced and which we all recognize."
Neither Lewis's statement nor Mackenzie's is of much help when one is
trying to approach the study of pain mechanisms scientifically. Defining
pain in terms of subjective personal experiences is as useful as telling a
blind man that everyone knows what the color red is.

Both Lewis and MacKenzie were right in acknowledging that the only
way we have to assess pain is through communication with other human
beings. As we will see later in the book, assessing the pain of others—
either humans or other animals—is not an easy task. When someone tells
us that he is in pain, all we can do is either believe him—or disbelieve
him; there is little else that would help us to measure other people's pain.
Pain is known to us by experience, as Lewis wrote; thus, if someone else
has an injury or a disease that we know is painful, we will believe that
person's pain. If we don't have a similar experience, we will just have to
accept that the other person is in pain. It is often said, humorously but
with a grain of truth, that there are two kinds of pain: mine, which is
always real, and yours, which is nothing but a lot of complaining. The
situation is even more complex when we deal with animals or with non-

communicating humans, such as babies. Do all animals feel pain? Can we assess pain in snails or chimpanzees? Is their pain experience similar to ours? And how about babies? We don't remember much of our early years. Can we then assume that there was no pain? Either we give animals and non-communicating humans the benefit of the doubt or we simply ignore their pain.

Sherrington's definition proposes an elegant separation between the protective-reflex component and the sensory perception of pain. The protective reflex includes a psychical adjunct that we call pain, but the two processes are separate. We can detect protective reflexes in all animals, from amebas to gorillas, and we can certainly see these reflexes in human babies and even in embryos. Sherrington used a special word to qualify the neural processes that deal with protective reflexes: *nociception*. This term refers to the processing by the brain of noxious events, such as injury or potential damage. It doesn't imply pain perception; on the contrary, it refers to the workings of the brain irrespective of whether or not there is pain perception. The idea of nociception allows scientists to study pain in anesthetized human beings and animals, in tissue cultures, or even in isolated cells. *Nociception* refers to the mechanisms that the brain uses to elaborate a response to an injury or to potential damage.

When we use the word *nociception*, we can separate the perception of pain from the chain of events triggered in the nervous system as a consequence of the injury. In the case of a burned finger, the study of nociception is the study of how high temperatures are signaled by nerve sensors in the skin of the finger, how these signals are transmitted to the brain, how nerve cells in the spinal cord and the brain react to these signals and communicate the injury-related messages to one another, and how the brain uses this information to move the muscles that withdraw the hand from the heat, or to change our blood pressure and respiration to adapt to the emergency, or even to help us to learn from this event for future reference. We can detect nociceptive activity in single cells, in isolated networks of cells, in all animals, and in anesthetized humans. We don't need consciousness to assess nociception, and thus we can study injury-related processes in the absence of pain perception.

Pain perception is identified in Sherrington's definition as a mental process, a psychical adjunct, added to a nociceptive mechanism. How and to whom we attribute this mental process depends on our social, religious, or scientific beliefs, and the key word here is certainly *belief*. Some people may argue that nociception and pain are entirely separate

processes, evidence of a dualism of body and soul. Others may regard pain as a final neural process triggered by nociception in a conscious individual. Which animal species are capable of adding pain perception to nociception can also be a matter of debate. Most of us would agree that pain perception, as we understand it in humans, probably is absent in amebas or snails, but not in dogs or chimpanzees. How we match pain and nociception is very much a question of personal values well beyond the realm of science, at least until we know a lot more about the workings of the brain.

Thinking of pain as the psychical adjunct of a protective reflex is a brilliant intellectual exercise that separates the two basic components of the process: the protective mechanism triggered by the brain and the mental process of sensory perception. We can apply the scientific method to the study of nociception in all biological systems from single cells to whole animals, and we can analyze in minute detail all the elements of a nociceptive or injury-detecting system. It is much more difficult, with our present knowledge of the brain, to assess pain perception in both humans and animals, and our interpretations are still colored by personal beliefs that are well beyond scientific inquiry. Although nociception is easily approached with the scientific method, understanding human pain is, at present, beyond that method's capabilities.

There is another serious limitation on the use of nociception as a scientific tool: no matter how much we know about the details of a certain nociceptive mechanism, we can't understand how that mechanism influences an individual's overall, and subjective, pain perception. How nociception leads to pain perception remains inaccessible to scientific inquiry. And there is another big caveat in Sherrington's definition. Many forms of pain are unrelated to protective reflexes, and their usefulness is questionable or even completely absent. The psychical adjunct of a protective reflex applies only to normal pain—the "good pain," the pain that protects us from injury. But what about the pain of disease? What about chronic pains, unrelated to any kind of injury, that make people's lives miserable for no reason? We must set good pain apart from evil pain. The two have very different meanings. Good pain is helpful and protective; evil pain is a curse. The brain mechanisms that mediate both forms of pain may even be different. The psychical adjunct of a protective-reflex definition doesn't apply to the pain of disease. Interestingly, Sherrington himself, later in life, recognized the limitations of his own definition. We will see at the end of this chapter how he dealt with this enigma.

To Serve And Protect: The Good Pain

If you add a few drops of acid to a small pond, or change the temperature of the water a little, the millions of single-cell creatures that inhabit the pond will quickly swim away from the unwelcome change. Gently poke a snail and it will retract inside its shell. Every vertebrate, from a fish to a gorilla, will react to injury or potential damage by withdrawing or moving away from the insult. Some will squeak, shout, or moan. All will learn very quickly that this wasn't a happy moment of their lives. Some animals have injury-inflicting weapons, such as big teeth, claws, horns, and stings, that they use very effectively to warn others to keep away from them or to entice them to do what they want. Protective reactions to injury and damage are among the oldest survival tricks in nature.

We humans have also developed pain perception as part of our protective equipment, and we believe that other species also have similar negative feelings associated with injury. Nerve cells capable of sensing tissue damage are one of the earliest developments of the nervous system, present in all living creatures from the simplest to the most complex. These sensors are connected with networks of cells in the brain that in turn move muscles to withdraw from a damaging stimulus and organize the rest of the control systems to adapt to the injury and help the organism to heal. An unpleasant sensation of pain is associated with this process to teach us that there was danger and to help us to learn not to do it again. This is the good pain, a normal component of our sensory repertoire, as useful as vision or hearing, something that we are all born with and that we cannot do without. Good pain protects us. It makes sure that we don't twist our joints or strain our muscles, that we don't grab a hot dish in the kitchen, that we don't bite our tongue. It serves us very well.

There has always been a scientific interpretation of pain that emphasizes its protective value. Sherrington's definition is a good example. René Descartes produced an earlier version in the seventeenth century. Descartes was a philosopher and a mathematician—he invented the Cartesian coordinates. He also wrote a book, titled *Traité de l'homme* (*Treatise of Man*), in which he described the human body as a machine. The Catholic Church regarded this approach as heretical because it seemed to deny the spiritual dimension of a human being. Descartes was well aware of this problem and applied two very important restrictions in his book. The first was a distinction between the material body and the spiritual soul, a strict dualism that allowed him to describe the

machinery of the human body under the control of a God-given and immortal soul. The second protection, just in case, was to request that the book not be published until after his death. The fact that the Catholic Church included all Descartes' writings in its list of forbidden books shows that his fears were not unfounded. *Traité de l'homme*, published in 1664 (14 years after his death), has remained a classic of both philosophy and biology.

One of the most enduring passages of Descartes' book is the one in which he describes how the nervous system deals with potential injury. It is accompanied by a beautiful drawing of a boy kneeling in front of a fire, his left foot dangerously close to the heat source. The drawing shows the pathways within the spinal cord and the brain that mediate the withdrawal reflex of the leg from the heat source. Descartes proposed that the particles of the fire excite the fine terminations of sensory nerves in

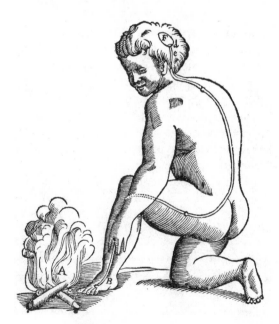

ainfi que tirant l'vn des bouts d'vne corde,
on fait fonner en mefme temps la cloche qui pend à
l'autre bout.

Figure 1.1
Pain as an alarm system. The figure and the line of text are from Descartes' *Traité de l'homme*, published in 1664. Pain is represented as a line that links the stimulus—the fire—with the brain. The quoted text from the book sums it up by saying that the pain sensation occurs "just as pulling one end of a cord one rings the bell that hangs at the other end."

the boy's foot and activate them to transmit this information all the way up to the brain, whereupon, reflected in the pineal gland in a mirror-like manner, they activate the motor nerves that pull the leg muscles so that the foot is withdrawn from the fire. What Descartes described was the *reflex arc*, a sensory-motor transformation that mediates the automatic withdrawal of a limb from a source of injury and that has retained the name *reflex* to this day as a reference to the mirror-like properties of this mechanism.

A very important aspect of Descartes' description is the way he refers to the process of pain perception in his model. Descartes thinks of pain as an alarm signal triggered by the heat burning the boy's foot and signaled by the transmission of the information from the foot to the brain. He describes the process in these words: "ainsi que tirant l'un des bouts d'une corde on fait sonner en même temps la cloche qui pend à l'autre bout" ("just as pulling one end of a cord one rings the bell that hangs at the other end"). It is hard to think of a better image of an alarm signal than that of a bell rung in the brain by the nerves that transmit the pain signal. This is the essence of the protective nature of the good pain: sensors all over the body can signal injury or potential damage and will transmit this information to the brain, where an alarm is triggered in the form of an unpleasant and powerful sensation of pain. The sensor pulls the cord and the pain bell rings in the brain.

Descartes' writings have been very influential in modern pain research. They stimulated the search for pain sensors in the periphery of the body and in internal organs, and they provided a philosophical background for the interpretation of brain function as a series of signals being transmitted through sensory and motor pathways. That this was a successful approach is demonstrated by the fact that many contemporary textbooks still present pain transmission as a linear pathway from the periphery of the body to the brain, very much like an alarm system. Comparing Descartes' drawing and a modern diagram of a pain pathway, one can see that the Cartesian approach is still very much in force 350 years later.

The protective nature of normal pain, the good pain, is dramatically demonstrated by what happens to those unfortunate people who are born without a pain system. Many people may think that being unable to feel pain would be a good thing, yet nothing is further from the truth. There are a number of very rare genetic disorders that affect the development of the neural systems that sense pain and that result in the birth of babies without a pain system and unable to feel any kind of pain.

Young children with congenital insensitivity to pain suffer all sorts of injuries. Often they bite their tongues or their fingers to the point of actually chewing the flesh. They have numerous infections, as their inflammatory reactions are also painless—sometimes even absent. Their joints are twisted and deformed. They sustain numerous injuries, including broken bones or major burns, and the injuries can be complicated by the fact that they never complain about these problems until they are apparent to caregivers. They often die young from complications of their injuries. A life without protective pain is not a happy life.

The conditions are extremely rare, but these patients are hard to forget. I have seen a case of congenital insensitivity to pain only once. A young girl, 12 or 13 years old, had gone to see a dermatologist because she had a bald patch on her head and, as adolescence developed, she wanted to so something about her appearance. Soon the dermatologist noticed a much bigger problem and called in specialists from the pain clinic. I joined them in examining the girl, who was a stunning example of the usefulness of protective pain. The bald patch on her head turned out to be a consequence of a major infection of the skull and the skin that she had when she was 3 years old. She had fallen off a swing in the playground but had continued to play even though, as was found later, she had fractured her skull. Eventually the fracture turned into an open infection, and she was treated, but by then her skin was seriously damaged; hence the bald patch. But that was not all. Half of her tongue was missing as a result of constant chewing when she was little. Most of her nails were also missing, as were the tips of her fingers, again as a consequence of repetitive chewing. She had sustained several limb fractures, most of them unnoticed until the bones were deformed. Her life had been a constant catalog of injuries of which she was never aware and which often developed into infections or deformities. She had survived by learning that there was a hostile and dangerous world out there of which she wasn't aware. To avoid injury, she had learned to interpret clues related to objects' shapes or other aspects of their appearances. Even though she couldn't feel any pain when cut or scalded, she knew that knives were sharp and that a boiling pot was hot. Her brain was desperately trying to help her survive by giving her clues other than pain about potential damage. I never saw the girl again, and I wonder if she managed to survive into adulthood without the protection of the good pain.

Virtually every case of this rare disease is published in the medical literature, and reading these stories gives you a good sense of how useful

the good pain is. Because these are genetic disorders, there are clusters of cases in the same family, and often patients help one another by sharing clues about the unfriendly world that exists beyond their ability to recognize injury. Their lives show how well the human brain can adapt to the most appalling situations. One young boy with congenital insensitivity to pain was reported to be able to feign pain after a tackle while playing soccer to ensure that the referee would call a foul against their opposing team. The survival capacity of the human brain is extraordinary.

The protective role of pain has often concealed that there is a lot more to pain than a simple alarm system that helps us to avoid injury. The Cartesian view of pain as an alarm bell and the idea that pain pathways carry injury-related information in a linear way to the brain for the purpose of protecting us from damage are correct, but they offer a very incomplete view of the whole range of pain mechanisms. Pain is a lot more than an alarm bell that rings in our brain when we touch something hot. Pain is also an emotion and an essential part of our memories. Pain molds people's personalities. It defines people's lives and sometimes ruins them. We will keep the good, protective nature of normal pain in mind, but we should also inquire about the other aspects of pain that make it a unique sensory and emotional experience far more complex than a simple alarm system.

A Passion of the Soul

Every schoolchild knows that there are five senses: hearing, sight, touch, smell, and taste. Pain is not in that list. The author of this most enduring list of human senses was the Greek philosopher Aristotle, who first included it in his book *De anima* (*On the Soul*), written around 350 BC. The fact that the Aristotelian idea of five senses is still prevalent today and the fact that pain hasn't made it onto the list show that the proposal is, if nothing else, persuasive. Any tenet that survives untouched more than 2,000 years must surely hold some truth.

Aristotle regarded as senses only those perceptions that could be associated with a particular sense organ: sight and the eye, hearing and the ear, smell and the nose, taste and the tongue, touch and the skin. He thought that pain wasn't linked to a particular sense organ but was associated with an extreme stimulation of any of the other senses. He viewed pain (and its opposite, pleasure) not as senses that give us information about the external world but as positive or negative engines of all human

behavior. He wrote: "We measure our actions by the rule of pleasure and pain. For this reason, then, our whole inquiry must be about these." Aristotle's views on pain, and on the meaning of pain, had a profound and enduring influence on Western philosophy even though he didn't focus on the sensory and protective aspects of pain. Aristotle was mostly concerned with the emotional and behavioral components of pain and pleasure. He thought that the two were the engines of all our actions. And he called them both "the passions of the soul."

The idea behind Aristotle's interpretation is that stimulation of any of the five senses gives us impressions of the outside world that we can use to inform us and guide our actions. But if any of the senses is stimulated with great intensity, or abnormally, or in a way that causes damage, the sensation changes to pain, and a "passion" or emotion moves us away from this feeling. Conversely, a pleasant stimulation of the senses gives us pleasure that acts as a positive drive of our behavior. The Aristotelian notion of the passions of the soul could be translated into modern language as "the emotions of our mind," meaning the positive and negative reinforcements that we associate with painful or pleasurable sensory perceptions and that shape our behavioral patterns. We certainly measure our actions by the rule of pleasure and pain. As the philosopher John Locke wrote in 1690: "Pleasure and pain and that which causes them, good and evil, are the hinges on which our passions turn."

These Aristotelian ideas aren't just philosophical curiosities. The notion that pain is not a sense, or at least that it differs from the other five senses, has survived to our day and has produced a line of scientific thought that considers pain to be the result of the pattern of stimulation of any sense organ. Some patterns can produce pleasurable sensations and others can lead to pain. What matters is not the activation of a specific sense organ but how that organ is stimulated. This has generated a scientific interpretation of pain, known as the *pattern theory*, that has challenged the mechanistic view of pain as an alarm line that connects the pain sensor in the skin with the ringing bell in the brain. As far as pain mechanisms are concerned, no two philosophies can be more contrary to each other than those of Descartes and Aristotle.

The Cartesian view of pain as an alarm system that accompanies a protective reflex generated the scientific approach known as the *specificity theory* of pain. The essence of this theory calls for the existence of pain sensors distributed throughout our body and connected to an alarm-signal-like pathway that transmits their messages to the brain, where a

pain bell rings. In neurobiological terms, the specificity theory compels us to look for sensory receptors in the skin and other tissues that are activated exclusively by injury or potential damage and for pain pathways in the spinal cord that transmit their signals to pain-processing centers in the brain.

On the other hand, the Aristotelian view of pain as a passion of the soul, a behavioral drive triggered by excessive stimulation of any sense organ, requires a very different neurobiological approach. We don't need specific pain receptors and alarm-like pathways; on the contrary, we need to look for patterns of activation of sense organs that we find unpleasant and for distributed processing of information by the brain. The pattern theory is therefore contrary to the existence of specific pain receptors and pain pathways and places its emphasis not on which systems are triggered by injury but on how these systems are activated. The Aristotelian and Cartesian philosophies produced two contradictory scientific theories of pain that in turn led to very different interpretations of how the brain deals with pain perception.

As usually happens in science when there are contradictory theories and interpretations, both the specificity theory and the pattern theory have elements of truth and serious deficiencies. As we will see in subsequent chapters, current knowledge of pain mechanisms is a synthesis of the two theories, the specificity interpretation being most adequate for the protective component of pain (the alarm-signal aspect) and the pattern theory providing a better explanation for the pathological aspects of pain perception (including chronic pain). We have come to understand that there isn't a single mechanism for all forms of pain. For a long time, pain was considered to be a single phenomenon, and therefore all that was needed to explain it was a single mechanism. Now we know that there is not one pain but many pains, and that various forms of pain may be the products of different brain mechanisms. Pain is indeed the psychical adjunct of a protective reflex and a powerful alarm signal that serves and protects us, but pain is also a passion of our souls, an emotion that drives our behavior, and in some cases, when unconnected with any protective role, a destructive curse.

One Pain, or Many Pains?

Suppose that you have just bought a new shirt. You carefully remove all the pins and try it on. Unfortunately, one of the pins has escaped your attention, and as you button up the shirt you feel a sharp pinprick in your

neck. You quickly remove the shirt and see the pin that is still attached to it. Wondering why shirts are packaged with so many pins, you remove the offending object and try the shirt on again. By now the sharp pain that told you about the omitted pin is gone. It was indeed pain, but hardly worth thinking about it. That was the good protective pain, the one we can't do without. We call it *nociceptive* pain.

Now suppose that you are hanging a picture in your study. You wanted to do this for quite some time, and today you decided to do it. You are in a hurry, and you don't concentrate on the job. You swing the hammer, trying to hit the nail. Instead you hit your thumb very hard. It hurts a lot, and the pain doesn't go away. If anything, it gets worse. After a few minutes your thumb is swollen and very painful. The pain will last for four or five days and will not go away until the thumb is no longer swollen and the wound has healed. This is also a protective pain: it forces you not to use your thumb while is being repaired. It also teaches you not to hammer your thumb again. But it is very different from the pain of a pinprick. We call it *inflammatory* pain.

There is a third and much nastier kind of pain. You have never felt it, but you know someone who has. A few years ago, a motorbike accident left him with a broken arm. The fracture severed a nerve in the arm, and he lost sensation in that arm for a few weeks. Then, after the fracture had healed and all was back to normal, he began to feel a burning pain in the area where he had previously lost sensation. This pain has little to do with the original accident, because the wound disappeared a long time ago. It is very intense, and it is there constantly. If anyone or anything touches the arm, it feels as if a red-hot bar is being pushed through the limb. A gentle breeze on the skin is like fire. Your friend protects the arm constantly to keep it from being touched. The pain is driving him crazy. It is a curse. We call this kind of pain *neuropathic*.

Nociceptive and inflammatory pains are normal pains. We all feel them, and we will continue to feel them occasionally for the rest of our lives. Nociceptive pain protects us from injury; inflammatory pain helps us to heal. Nociceptive pain is seldom a cause for concern; we don't go to see a physician because we have felt a pinprick or touched something hot. Such pain is normal but not clinically relevant. On the other hand, inflammatory pain can be very intense — think of a tooth extraction — and we want to reduce it. Inflammatory pain is normal but is also clinically relevant. Things can go wrong if inflammatory pain becomes long lasting, maintained by a persistent inflammatory condition such as chronic

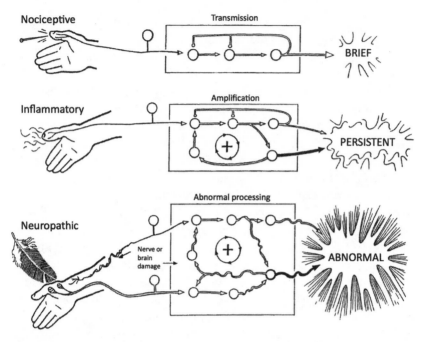

Figure 1.2
The three kinds of pain—nociceptive, inflammatory, and neuropathic—and the relationship
between the stimulus and the pain produced in each of them: brief in response to a simple
injury, persistent as a consequence of inflammation, and abnormal as a result of damage
to a nerve or to the brain. The circuits are idealized diagrams of the underlying mechanisms:
a simple transmission chain in the case of nociceptive pain, an amplification mechanism
for inflammatory pain, abnormal processing mechanisms for neuropathic pain. Adapted
from F. Cervero and J. M. A. Laird, "One Pain or Many Pains?" *News in Physiological Sci-
ences* 6 (1991): 268–273.

arthritis. A constant and painful inflammation is a disease in its own right,
not a helpful and protective process.

Neuropathic pain is always caused by a disease of the nervous system.
It is definitely not normal, and fortunately many of us will go throughout
our entire lives without ever feeling it. Neuropathic means that the
nervous system is damaged. For a variety of reasons, including trauma,
degeneration, and metabolic alterations, the machinery in our nerves and
brains that we use to detect normal pain goes wrong and the association
between injury and pain is lost. Pain is felt in the absence of injury or is
triggered by processes that ordinarily don't cause it (for example, touch
or cold). Neuropathic pain has a particularly nasty quality. It feels like a
burn or an electric shock, and it is very difficult to treat. Neuropathic

pain is abnormal and very much clinically relevant. A great deal of current research into pain mechanisms is directed at unraveling the mysteries of neuropathic pain and at developing more effective treatments for it.

The main feature that differentiates nociceptive, inflammatory, and neuropathic pain from one another is that in each of the three kinds there is a different relationship between injury and pain. Normal forms of pain show close and direct association. In the case of nociceptive pain, the association is immediate: a brief, minor injury leads to a brief, minor pain. It is the simplest kind of alarm system, the best example of the psychical adjunct of a protective reflex. Inflammatory pain maintains a relationship between the originating injury and the pain—you hit your thumb and it hurts—but there is a temporal dissociation in that the injury lasts for a second and the pain for four or five days. The distinctive feature of inflammatory pain is that the injury causes tissue damage, which in turn triggers an inflammatory process that repairs the wound. The inflammation causes the nervous system to move to a more excitable state for the duration of the healing process, and this amplifies the signals from the inflamed part of the body. The amplification contributes to the high intensity of the pain and prolongs its duration beyond the moment of injury while maintaining, throughout the healing process, a close relationship between injury and pain.

The destruction of the normal relationship between injury and pain is what makes neuropathic pain truly dreadful. Your arm, your leg, or your back hurts in the absence of injury. You can't find an explanation for this pain. Types of stimulation that normally don't cause pain, such as touch or cold, now produce excruciating pain. In some cases pain is felt in limbs that are no longer there, as in the case of phantom-limb pain that develops after an amputation. There is simply no rational explanation for this hideous pain that makes your life unbearable. Losing the normal relationship between injury and pain transforms the beneficial, protective alarm system into an evil enemy.

John Bonica, an American anesthesiologist who pioneered the development of specialized pain clinics and became the founder of modern pain medicine, explained the difference between the good protective pain and the awful pathological pain eloquently: "Whereas acute symptomatic pain serve the useful purpose of warning, chronic pain is a malefic force which imposes severe emotional, physical, and economic stresses on the patient." Thanks to Bonica's graphic qualification of chronic pain as a malefic force and to the focus on the personal and social

suffering it causes, we now regard chronic pain as a disease in its own right.

If there are so many different forms of pain, some good and protective and others negative and malefic, and if some pains are helpful but others destructive, can we think of all forms of pain as products of a single, unique brain mechanism? This question may sound very simplistic, but only in the last two or three decades has the distinction between normal and abnormal pain been considered fundamental to the understanding of pain mechanisms. We now know that there are many forms of pain, some elements of the normal sensory repertoire and others products of a damaged neurological mechanism. The brain systems that mediate the pain of a pinprick can't be the same ones that maintain phantom-limb pain or the pain of trigeminal neuralgia. Different forms of pain are mediated by different brain mechanisms. Some forms of neuropathic pain are attributable to the transformation of a normal nociceptive process into a source of spontaneous or abnormal pain. For instance, one consequence of sustaining an injury is the development of an increased sensitivity to pain around the area of damage, a normal feature of noci- ceptive and inflammatory pain. But in some pathological cases in which the nervous system itself is the source of the damage, this enhanced pain sensitivity may be triggered in the absence of an originating injury or with a disproportionate intensity. Neuropathic pain is a pathological consequence of the neurological damage, and what we see in the patient is the expression of a normal pain mechanism triggered in the absence of injury. In other cases, the mechanisms that mediate inflammatory or neuropathic pain are very different from those set in motion during nociceptive pain. The simple Cartesian model of a linear pathway that carries pain messages from the skin to the brain can explain the pain of a pinprick but fails to offer a possible mechanism for inflammatory pain. And there is also the possibility, supported by plenty of experimental evidence, that damage to the nervous system can set in motion new mechanisms and processes different from those that mediate normal forms of pain. There are many kinds of pain, there are many kinds of pain mechanisms, and not all pain mechanisms are responsible for all kinds of pain.

A Biological Enigma

I opened this chapter with Charles Sherrington's magnificent definition of pain as the psychical adjunct of a protective reflex, and I have been

adding caveat after caveat to it to the point that we should ask ourselves if the definition is useful at all. Pain is a protective sensation, of course, but not always. Pain is not just a sense; it is also an emotion, a passion of the soul, and pain is not a unique process anyway. There are many forms of pain, some useful and others useless. Some kinds of pain are inexplicable in evolutionary terms, and they become malefic forces that disable the patients to the point of making their lives miserable.

To be fair to Sherrington, he was also aware that his description of pain had some limitations. He wrote his original definition in 1900, when he was 43 years of age. Forty years later, in 1940, he added some reflections about pain in a letter to his former pupil John F. Fulton, then a professor of physiology at Yale University: "Pain remains a biological enigma—so much of it useless, a mere curse." There is very little left of the protective reflex in these words. What we have instead is a very explicit revelation of human nature. At 43, pain is indeed, for most people, a helpful consequence of a protective reflex. But at age 83, when Sherrington was frail, old, and sick, he could see that much of his own pain was useless, a mere curse, and that from a mechanistic point of view there was still much to be learned about this biological enigma.

One of the products of John Bonica's enormous energy was the founding, in 1973, of the International Association for the Study of Pain (IASP). This association has became the prime professional organization for scientists and clinicians interested in pain and has produced a nomenclature of pain terms and conditions to help professionals from many disciplines to communicate effectively. High on the agenda of IASP's taxonomy committee was to come up with a definition of pain. The result, first published in 1979, is still the accepted definition of pain today: "an unpleasant sensory and emotional experience associated with actual or potential tissue damage, or described in terms of such damage." The taxonomy committee needed a few more words than the seven Sherrington used, but the definition covers all the various aspects of pain. It is an experience, both sensory and emotional, and always unpleasant. This definition goes well beyond a psychical adjunct and deals with both the Aristotelian approach and the Cartesian approach. It regards pain as associated with, not caused by, actual or potential tissue damage. These are very carefully measured words, and there is no mention of protection. The final few words take care of abnormal and pathological pains. Even when there is no actual injury, pain is felt as if it there were one.

Armed with an accurate definition of pain, and with the knowledge that pain is not a simple sensation but a complex and enigmatic experi-

ence with many dimensions, I will now attempt to discuss the intricacies of the bits and pieces of the brain that deal with the signaling of injury and whose activity lead to the perception of pain. And we need to keep in mind what one of my medical students wrote in an essay on pain many years ago: "We have never understood pain. It has been an obsession of religion, literature, philosophy and science, called at times an evil and at others a punishment for evil. Pain is physical and pain is emotional, pain is inevitable and pain can be overcome. Now pain is in the hands of the physiologists and we are still in the dark."

Chances are that while you are reading this book someone somewhere is doing a tail-flick test. This is an experimental procedure aimed at measuring pain in laboratory rats and mice to test the analgesic properties of drugs and other compounds. It is the most popular method to assess pain ever developed and in view of the large number of research laboratories and drug companies interested in pain mechanisms it is likely that a tail-flick test is in progress at this very moment somewhere in the world.

Two American scientists, Fred D'Amour and Donn Smith, developed the tail-flick test in 1941. They described the method and their initial experimental findings in a short research paper that is a real gem. They recognized the difficulties of measuring pain in laboratory animals and the need to develop simple and quantitative methods for the testing of new analgesic drugs. With charming candor, they criticized previous rudimentary techniques based on piling weights on a cat's tail, heating a rat's skin with hot water, or applying electric shocks of 100–800 volts to a rat's scrotum. Their goal was to find a stimulus that was painful, brief, easy to deliver, not very damaging, and easy to quantify. They settled for the application of controlled radiant heat to the tip of a rat's tail. They also needed to determine an end-point reaction to this stimulus that would be clearly related to the stimulus, would show little variability, and would be sensitive to known analgesic drugs. They decided to measure the time it took for the rat to flick its tail and remove it from the heat source.

The method couldn't be simpler. A rat is held on a flat board and its tail is laid straight on a groove on the board. Then a light bulb is focused on the tip of the tail and a stopwatch is started. The power of the lamp is set so that the rat will flick its tail and remove it from the heat source about five seconds after the start of the test. If a test drug is given to the

rat and the time to trigger the tail flick is prolonged beyond five seconds, the interpretation is that the drug has analgesic properties. D'Amour and Smith tried a number of snake and spider venoms, found no change in tail-flick time, and concluded that those compounds weren't analgesics. Then they tried several opiates—morphine, codeine, and heroin—and observed a strong and reproducible increase in the tail-flick time that was directly related to the dose of the opiate given to the rat. The greater the dose, the longer it took for the rat to flick its tail. The tail-flick test of analgesia had just been born.

The test was subsequently refined and a good deal of technology was added to it. Several rats or mice can be tested at the same time. Computers (which also control various sources of radiant heat, including sophisticated light beams) trigger time-measuring devices and lasers and, at the same time, measure the tail flick automatically with movement sensors. The heat source has a safety device that cuts off the stimulus if the animal doesn't move its tail at all. D'Amour and Smith referred to this immobile state as one of *complete analgesia* and, in their characteristically direct style, described this loss of reaction as follows: "The animal makes no movement of the tail whatever even though it is being burned to a crisp." To appease the alarmed reader, they added: "It is, of course, not necessary to burn it to that extent, a white blistering appearance being sufficient."

The tail-flick test spread through research laboratories and pharmaceutical companies like wildfire. It is easy to do and easy to standardize, can be done by research personnel with relatively little training, is reliable, shows little variability, is very sensitive to known analgesics, and produces numerical values that can be analyzed statistically to quantify the analgesic power of a test compound. It is a godsend for people who want an easy way to measure pain—or so they think—and aren't very worried about what they are really measuring. Soon other methods based on similar approaches were developed. A variation of the original tail-flick test is based on dipping the tail of a rat or a mouse in a hot bath at 50 degrees centigrade and measuring how long it takes the animal to remove the tail from the water. The related *hot-plate test* calls for placing animals on a platform preheated to 45–50°C and measuring how long it takes them to lick their paws or jump about. Other methods have proposed the use of mechanical stimuli, such as pinching a tail or applying pressure to a paw. All are based, one way or another, on applying a brief, acute, and quantified painful stimulus to a body part of an animal and measuring how long it takes the animal to remove the body part from the source of the stimulus.

The tail-flick test, like the other related tests, measures a simple reflex: the short-lived withdrawal reaction to a brief stimulus that may cause pain. The relationship between this fast and automatic reflex and the complexities of clinically relevant pain is, at best, tenuous. It is important to state, for the record, that D'Amour and Smith included a big disclaimer in their paper: "The subject of analgesia is a complex one and we are here using the term *analgesia* as synonymous with loss of reaction to pain merely for convenience sake." And they added: "No claim is made that the method is capable of determining the analgesic power of drugs when deep-seated, continuous pain is involved." It is a pity that these words of caution were soon forgotten for the sake of expediency.

What the tail-flick test measures is a sensory-motor transformation that takes place mostly in the spinal cord. Injury sensors in the skin are activated by heating the tail and send information to the brain. When the information reaches the spinal cord, it is distributed through various pathways, including one within the spinal cord that connects with the spinal neurons that move the relevant muscles away from the source of the stimulus. The tail flick is the expression of a simple spinal reflex. Obviously these reflexes, like the entire brain, are affected by drugs that change the excitability of the nervous system, and therefore there is a weak relationship between the strength of a reflex and the perception of the stimulus that triggered the reflex. The spinal reflex is also under the control of higher centers of the brain, and if we modify their activity it follows that the reflex is also modified. But the perception of pain will occur only when the information from the injury sensors in the tail reaches the brain. We know that the two processes, the motor reflex and the sensory perception, are mediated by different systems and can easily be dissociated. A rat with poor motor coordination as a result of administration of a test drug will give abnormal results in a tail-flick test even though its pain perception may remain intact. Therefore, even for the short-lived reaction to an acute and brief injury such as that of the tail flick, it is not possible to equate reaction time with pain perception. If we add the complexities of chronic pain, or those of the pain produced by disease, and the emotional and affective dimensions of persistent pain in humans, it is harder to associate a tail flick with pain perception. Ultimately pain is all in the brain, so when measuring pain we need fewer tails and more heads.

The main problem with the tail-flick test and other similar procedures is that they are used for purposes other than those for which they were originally developed. To be fair, these simplistic methods of pain assessment in experimental animals can be useful if we are aware of what are

we measuring. The reaction time of a spinal reflex may be indicative of how quickly injury-related information is transmitted through the spinal cord and toward the brain. Changes in brain processing may also be reflected in the control that the brain exerts over spinal reflexes. An analgesic drug acting in the brain can also induce changes in the motor reaction to a brief injury. There is some information about pain and analgesia that can be extracted from a judicious use of tail-flick tests. We should not forget that the most important piece of equipment of any scientific test is the experimenter's own brain.

Nothing exemplifies the difficulty of measuring pain in humans and animals better than the tail-flick test. On the one hand, we need to apply scientific rigor to objective measurements that can be quantified; hence the controlled light sources, the accurate time keeping, and the clear-cut endpoints. On the other hand, we are dealing with pain—one of the most complex and subjective of all our sensations and emotions, and one that is always colored with personal, social, and biological factors. The dilemma is this: we need to simplify in order to measure accurately, but if we simplify too much we depart from the very object of our study. If you would rather not be bothered with these inconveniences, or if you are in a hurry to test your experimental compound, the tail-flick test is the one for you. But you must be aware that you will not be dealing with the intricacies of clinically relevant human pain.

For a long time, physicians and scientists have been trying to quantify the pain of their patients and striving to develop reliable methods for measuring human and animal pain. Tests and methods based on objective and quantifiable measurements have been developed, but the simplest and most robust of them, such as the tail-flick test, are far from reproducing the conditions of clinically relevant pain.

Can we objectively measure pain in our fellow human beings? How accurately can we assess pain perception and pain relief? Can we measure or assess pain in animals? Can we develop experimental methods that make it practicable to study pain and to discover new analgesic drugs for the treatment of clinically relevant conditions? And can we measure pain in others and still honor our ethical obligations to the subjects of our studies, be they humans or animals?

Measuring Pain in Humans

Low-back pain is the most frequent kind of pain. More than 80 percent of people older than 30 years have experienced or will experience low-

back pain, and for many of them it becomes a chronic ailment. The prevalence of this kind of pain is only slightly less than that of the common headache. Low-back pain is also the greatest cause of disability and of loss of working days. Jobs that require standing for a long time or involve lifting a load cannot be carried out if you experience low-back pain. Sometimes even sitting down for a few minutes triggers the pain. In the United States alone the annual cost of low-back pain exceeds 50 billion dollars, and in countries with socialized medical care the disability costs generated by low-back pain are escalating to a point where the entire system of workers' compensation is endangered.

Low-back pain is also a mysterious condition. The pain is localized in the lower back and often radiates down the legs. It is associated with muscle spasms and contractures, but the actual cause is not always obvious. Sometimes, but by no means always, it is attributable to a displacement of the cushions that separate the vertebrae and give elasticity to the vertebral column: the intervertebral discs. Herniated discs compress or pinch the nerves entering and leaving the spinal cord and cause pain that irradiates to the point of origin of the compressed nerve. In a few patients it is possible to find radiological evidence of damage to or degeneration of the discs or the vertebrae, but in many others, who complain of considerable pain, nothing abnormal is detected in the vertebral column. There is often little correlation between obvious signs of muscle, bone, or joint damage and the intensity of low-back pain. In some cases nothing at all is found to explain this intense pain in the lower area of the back. To make matters worse, there are also people with extensive radiological evidence of damage to the joints in the vertebral column who feel no back pain at all.

Yet patients who complain of pain in their backs are likely to lose working days, claim disability, and eventually get early retirement or compensation, all as consequences of a debilitating chronic disease that, in many cases, doesn't show any objective signs of damage. Is this pain real? Can we measure objectively whether these patients are truly in pain? In view of the economic and social costs, it is understandable that insurance companies and government health services demand objective signs of the disease that is causing the pain.

What physicians and insurance companies would like to have is a *dolorimeter*—a device that would accurately measure whether a person is in pain and how much pain he or she feels. We have thermometers and blood-pressure meters to obtain objective measurements of the signs of disease, but when it comes to pain all we have is what the patients tell

us. And it is one thing to sympathize with our patients and another to use scarce resources, spend large amounts of money, and remove people from gainful employment for diseases whose main or only symptom is a verbal report of pain. Can we measure pain objectively?

There have been many attempts at building dolorimeters, but the results have been disappointing. Most of the instruments measure pain thresholds and pain tolerance rather than absolute pain sensation. Even more difficult is to assess objectively whether a pain is real or imaginary. One of the first dolorimeters was designed more than 50 years ago by a group of American pain doctors and scientists led by the physicist James Hardy and the neurologist Harold Wolff. Light generated by a 1,000-watt lamp, focused with a lens, and passed through a shutter that opened for 3 seconds was projected on a small area of a subject's skin that had been blackened to reduce reflection. The intensity of the light, and hence the heat produced, was progressively increased until the subject reported pain. Then the instrument was focused on a radiometer to measure the amount of light that had generated the pain sensation. Measurements were made in several areas of the body, and the pain threshold and the maximum pain sensation reported by the subject were noted. Analgesics (including aspirin and morphine) and other procedures (including drinking alcohol) were then tried on the subject to check whether they raised the pain threshold and increased tolerance as measured with the dolorimeter. These studies demonstrated, among many other things, that a couple of stiff drinks raised the pain threshold to a level equivalent to that produced by a standard dose of codeine, thus giving scientific credibility to a method of administering pain relief in harsh environments often depicted in Hollywood movies.

Hardy and Wolff generated a large quantity of carefully measured numerical data on pain thresholds and responses. They came up with a pain scale based on the pain thresholds of volunteers (who included Hardy and Wolff) and the amount of radiant heat generated by their instrument. They divided the range into a ten-point scale of pain measured in units calls *Dols* (from *dolor*, Latin for "pain").

However, Hardy and Wolff ran into difficulty when they tried to use their Dol scale to measure clinically relevant pain. After asking patients to rate their disease-produced pain by reference to the pain generated with the dolorimeter, they attempted to establish a quantitative scale of pain measured in Dols. Unfortunately, this approach did not produce consistent and reproducible results, and eventually it was abandoned.

This initial attempt has not been the only one at designing a pain-measuring machine. Other scientists and physicians have also tried to induce controlled and brief pain using stimuli generated by radiant heat, pressure, lasers, and other devices. Not one of these attempts has resulted in a useful machine that is used regularly in a clinical setting. The main reason for this is that very controlled and quantitative methods of inducing pain experimentally do not reproduce clinically-relevant pain conditions. We can indeed measure very accurately the pain response to a controlled brief stimulus, but that doesn't help in assessing the magnitude of disease-induced or chronic pains. In 1937 the French surgeon René Leriche published a book titled *La chirurgie de la douleur* in which he argued passionately that there was a fundamental difference between *la douleur laboratoire* (laboratory pain) and *la douleur maladie* (disease pain), the former being, in his view, of little use in evaluating the latter.

Nevertheless, attempts at quantifying human pain, especially the pain of disease, have produced a very useful tool that is currently the main, if not the only, instrument used in hospitals and clinics to evaluate pain in patients: the *visual analogue scale* (VAS). The VAS is a logical offshoot of the Dol scale of Hardy and Wolff. It also uses a ten-point scale to rate pain, but it requires no complex machinery or sophisticated equipment. All you need is a pencil, a sheet of paper, and the ability to communicate with your patient.

The VAS is essentially a straight line drawn on a paper. Purists require that the line be exactly 10 centimeters long, but that isn't always neces-sary. At one end it is labeled 0, at the other end 10—or sometimes 100. Between the two ends there are marks at regular intervals that can also be labeled 1, 2, 3, . . . (or, with a 100-point scale, 10, 20, 30, . . .). The clini-cian simply asks the patient to rate the pain, with 0 meaning no pain at all and 10—or 100—meaning the maximum pain imaginable. That is all. Amazingly, the subjective ratings of pain by individual patients are very

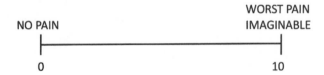

Figure 2.1
Measuring pain: the visual analogue scale (VAS). The line should be 10 centimeters long. The subject rates the pain by placing a mark on the line at the appropriate point according to the labels at each extreme. Pain is then measured on a scale from 0 to 10.

consistent over long periods of time. For instance, after surgery you may want to chart the evolution of postoperative pain and adjust an analgesic schedule. If you take VAS readings at regular time intervals, you will immediately see the effectiveness of your treatment. The same is true if you are testing a new analgesic drug in volunteers or patients. The verbal reports of the subjects, expressed numerically and graphically on a simple line, generate accurate, reproducible, and quantifiable results.

Technology couldn't be kept out of the VAS, and many variations have been produced. The straight line drawn on a paper has been replaced with computer screens, hand-held electronic devices and rows of lamps and electronic controls that output the values selected by the patients to computers that then store and analyze the data. But ultimately all this boils down to a line and a numerical scale on which patients rate their pain.

Sometimes images are added to the VAS—a smiley face at the 0 point and progressively pained facial expressions leading to a face showing extreme pain at the scale's maximum point. "Face-based" VAS is very useful for testing young children and others who can't communicate well with words or numbers, as well as in multilingual settings. Other variations include sliders over pieces of cardboard or plastic and every imaginable way of expressing a numerical value on a scale. But in essence, any VAS is just a line and a numerical scale.

Measuring pain with VAS is almost an art form. The standard VAS is a numerical scale with the words "no pain" at one end and "worst imaginable pain" at the other. But there are also more elaborate scales that test the distress caused by pain using a scale of words such as *annoying*, *dreadful*, and *agonizing*, and there are some that focus on the emotional aspect of pain by using words that are related to the pleasant or unpleasant components of the sensations. With a VAS, various aspects of pain perception, from sensory to emotional, can be assessed using words that qualify the pain attribute that is being measured. What is remarkable is the consistency of the values obtained from the same patient over time or from populations of patients with a similar condition or treatment.

The use of visual analogue scales to measure various aspects of pain evolved into a more complex tool that is recognized worldwide as the best instrument for a comprehensive assessment of pain: the McGill Pain Questionnaire. Developed by Ronald Melzack at McGill University in the 1970s, it is based on the selection by the patients of the adjectives that best describe their pains. All aspects of pain sensation are considered, including intensity, unpleasantness, change with time, and type

of pain. The questionnaire includes 20 groups of words that qualify all aspects of pain with 80 adjectives — *flickering, pulsating, shooting, throbbing, lacerating, burning, aching, sore, unbearable,* and so on. Numerical scores are calculated to assess the sensory, emotional, and cognitive aspects of the pain condition. The questionnaire extracts a comprehensive chart of the pain as felt by the patient and offers diagnostic clues as to the causes of the pain based on the specific questionnaire profile of a certain pain condition. It turns out that we all use similar adjectives when qualifying similar types of pain; for instance, inflammatory pain is often described as pulsating or throbbing, and neuropathic pain is often felt as burning or shooting.

Over the years, the McGill Pain Questionnaire has been translated into virtually every major language. Translations require careful validation to make sure that the various adjectives have the same meanings in each language and to take cultural variations into account. Unfortunately, proper administration of the questionnaire requires considerable time, and this limits its use in busy clinical settings. There is also an abbreviated version that reportedly produces satisfactory results and takes less time to complete.

The VAS and the McGill Pain Questionnaire are products of a very practical — and very old — approach to the assessment of subjective feelings: listen to what the patients say. They focus on the important components of a subjective report, and they extract data that can be quantified and analyzed. They also reveal that studying verbal communication between patients and their caregivers is the best way to analyze a problem as complex as pain. The Spanish physician Gregorio Marañón used to say that a doctor's most useful diagnostic instrument is a chair, which is very true and often forgotten in present-day medical practice.

The difficulty of assessing pain objectively and the development of techniques based on verbal reports and visual scales haven't discouraged people from seeking objective methods of measuring pain in humans. The search for a perfect dolorimeter is still on. To avoid the subjective element of a verbal report, the ideal method should be based on the association of the pain reported by the patients with an objective recording of patterns of brain activity thus showing that the pain is real by obtaining a brain signature that correlates exclusively with the perception of pain. It would be even better if the machine would also indicate the intensity of the pain.

One approach is to record the electrical signals generated by the brain and relate their patterns of activity to a specific pain state. This can be

done by recording the electrical activity of the whole brain by means of an electroencephalogram or by recording the electrical activity of specific areas of the brain under provoked stimulation in the form of evoked electrical potentials. Recordings from pain patients are then compared with those of normal volunteers. In certain cases it is possible to detect anomalies in the recordings from pain patients but it is difficult to determine whether they are due to abnormal pain perception or to a brain dysfunction caused by an underlying neurological disorder. The electrical activity of individual neurons in the brain and of single nerve fibers in peripheral nerves can also be recorded with very fine electrodes, but this requires considerable instrumentation and can't be done routinely. Variations in the electrical activity of individual neurons may be related to aspects of brain processing other than sensory perception, and all we can discern from these recordings is that the activity of individual neurons may be abnormal. To establish an unequivocal correlation between a specific pattern of neuronal electrical activity and a specific pain perception is still a challenge.

Progress has also been made with the use of brain imaging. There has been a revolution in the use of sophisticated imaging of brain activity, both when the subjects are at rest and when they are performing various tasks. Many different methods are used to obtain maps of brain activity related to specific forms of induced stimulation or even to mental or emotional states. The brains of volunteers and patients are scanned when they are at rest or when they are performing tasks, rating evoked pain sensations, or even when they are anticipating the application of a painful stimulus. Studies have also been made of brain activation during emotional states associated with pain perception, including empathy with loved ones and fear of impending pain. Brain maps are being put together showing the various regions that are activated by painful stimuli and the sequence and intensity of the activation. These studies are still in their early stages, but the multitude of probes that are being developed to image brain functions and the data obtained so far have shown a promising path in our search for the perfect dolorimeter. In the not-too-distant future, we may be able to assess objectively, by looking at a functional brain map, whether a person is in pain and how much pain he or she is feeling.

Measuring Pain in Animals

An interesting feature of human nature is the capacity to project our feelings and emotions onto other species. Walt Disney and other cartoon-

ists have made very successful careers gratifying our innate empathy with animals by creating a whole cast of cheeky mice, foolish cats, lovable ducks, charming dogs, huggable bears, and even glamorous skunks, all of whom are as human as any of us. We transfer our feelings of pain and suffering to battery-caged hens, chased foxes, overworked donkeys, and force-fed geese. This is a peculiar and exclusively human trait. Real crocodiles and lions don't worry at all about the prey they kill and chew, including the occasional human being.

Why do we care so much about the pain that species other than our own might feel? The explanation is ethics. We have an innate need to organize our behavior with a set of rules that govern everything we do individually and collectively. Human behavior is led by a strong element of morality that, among many other things, controls our relations with other species. Ethical rules are universal at any point in time, but over the course of history they have varied greatly. Not very long ago, the most powerful nations in the world engaged in slavery and transferred large populations of human beings from Africa to the Americas. This was acceptable at the time, and some of these nations continued to practice racial segregation until very recently. Nowadays slavery and racial discrimination are abhorred by the very nations that previously practiced it, and this set of principles is imposed on the rest of the world. Right now we are in the middle of a passionate debate that may change our moral attitude toward other species. Central to the debate is the need to assess whether animals feel pain and whether they are capable of suffering.

Animals are used for all sorts of activities, some of which are essential for our survival (e.g., food and clothing) and some of which are superfluous (e.g., the use of animals in sports and entertainment). We force animals to work for us in agriculture and transportation, not to mention sniffing drugs, controlling crowds, ceremonial parades, and even warfare. Sometimes we use animals just for our own gratification, as when we keep them as pets. And we also use animals as experimental subjects in scientific research to find about our own biology. The current moral attitude toward the use of animals is based on a self-imposed obligation to use them humanely and responsibly while taking into account their capacity for pain and suffering. We don't attribute to animals the same fundamental rights that we attribute to ourselves (life, liberty, and the pursuit of happiness); if we did, we wouldn't be able to keep them in captivity or use them for food. But we do impose on ourselves a moral obligation to treat them humanely and tend to their needs. And that includes assessing their pain.

Is the pain experience of an animal similar to that of a human? Are animals capable of suffering as a consequence of the activities that we force on them? When we are engaged in pain research using experimental animals, the answers to these questions develop into a circular argument: we use animals to find out about pain mechanisms because they must have some sort of pain system similar to ours. If they didn't feel pain at all, their use in pain research wouldn't be justified. How much pain they feel and whether their experience is similar or identical to ours are the crucial questions. The practices of the veterinary profession are a very interesting indicator of our attitude toward animal pain. Widespread use of anesthetics in animal surgery and of analgesics in postoperative periods and control of painful procedures in abattoirs and in everyday farming activities are all indicators of a growing concern among veterinarians about minimizing and treating animal pain. Although there are no clear-cut answers to questions about the pain felt by animals in industrial environments, our society, led in this case by veterinarians, is moving toward giving the benefit of the doubt to the animals and reducing their pain.

From a scientific point of view the question of animal pain has two very different aspects. The first is the existence in animals of neurological mechanisms that can detect injury, or potential damage, and trigger actions aimed at preventing or reducing the injury. This is pure nociception, in the Sherringtonian sense, and is very much amenable to scientific inquiry down to the unraveling of the cells and molecules involved in the protective process. Injury-detection mechanisms exist in every animal from amebas to chimpanzees. The challenge is to extract those features of the mechanism that are common to various species, including humans. The second aspect of animal pain is much more complex and therefore harder to approach. We know that animals can have injury-detection mechanisms similar to ours, but do they have a pain experience similar to ours too? This question is almost impossible to answer. The only methods we have of assessing the pain experience of our own fellow human beings are based on verbal communication. Trying to judge and measure pain experiences in animals also requires some form of communication.

We are still far from having an objective method for the measurement of human pain. How, then, can we measure the pain of species with which we can't communicate? In 1942, proposing a very subjective definition of pain, Thomas Lewis wrote that "pain is known to us by experience and described by illustration." It isn't surprising that when discussing

animal pain Lewis stated that "there are no reliable and usable indices of pain in animals" and that "we have no knowledge of pain beyond that derived from human experience." In other words, all we can do is to attribute a sensory component of pain to the reactions we observe in animals when they are subjected to stimuli that we find painful. We touch something hot and we withdraw quickly from the heat source while feeling a sensation of burning pain. Therefore, the assumption goes, if we apply heat to an animal and it withdraws quickly from the heat source, the animal must have felt burning pain.

To assess pain in a laboratory animal, we measure its withdrawal reaction and assume that the avoidance of further exposures to the stimulus indicate that these are unpleasant experiences for the animal. But we can't know whether the animal actually felt a sensation identical to that that we would feel under the same circumstances. What we measure, in an experimental animal, are the reactions of withdrawal, avoidance, and rejection of the stimulus. To interpret them as surrogates for a pain sensation is not a problem-free approach. Behavioral responses to injury are present in most animal species, including invertebrates, but it is difficult to believe that a bee, a squid, or a fish has the same pain experience as a mouse, a dog, a chimpanzee, or a human being. Sherrington put it this way: "In all this experimental work on animals the observer has to work through signs of subjective states incomparably inferior in most instances to the verbal communication with an intelligent human being."

Virtually all laboratory models of experimental pain in animals are based on analyses of their behavioral responses to stimuli that are painful and unpleasant to humans. The methods require that the behavior be a positive one—that is, that the animal *do* something, such as move away, take some action, change its posture, or simply flick its tail. An animal that freezes when in pain doesn't generate an active behavior that can be assessed. Therefore, the two basic elements of every animal pain test are a controlled painful stimulus and the detection of a positive behavioral reaction. The complexity of the technique is directly related to the meaning of the relevant pain mechanism, and so we can study anything from a very simple reflex to a comprehensive behavioral pattern.

We use many animal models of pain, some simple and some more complex. At one end of the spectrum are techniques that measure reaction times to a brief and not very intense painful stimulus. These include the tail-flick test and similar techniques using hot plates and other such devices. Although these techniques are easy to use and are somewhat related to the processing of acute and mild pain, they are unlikely to give

us much information about the mechanisms of chronic and persistent pain that are much more relevant to human pain. Another group of techniques commonly used are those directed at exploring a mechanism involved in the processing of pain. For instance, we may be interested in understanding how pain sensors or nociceptors react to various forms of stimulation in normal conditions and in the presence of an inflammation. This will give us information about how pain signals are sent to the brain during an inflammatory process, and that information will help us to develop combined anti-inflammatory and analgesic drugs. Controlled inflammations of peripheral organs or tissues are induced in experimental animals to study the process of inflammation as well as the overall behavioral reaction to the injury that causes the inflammatory response. Using these procedures, it is possible to study how the brain reacts to a pain-producing process and to identify the molecular mechanisms involved in the pain reaction.

At the next level of complexity of animal models of pain are those that reproduce as closely as possible the diseases that induce pain in humans, such as a peripheral neuropathy, a joint inflammation, or a renal colic. In these cases it is important that the symptoms observed be similar to those of the disease under study, and that the treatments developed using this approach also work to treat the pain of the pathological condition. Such studies are difficult to do, and not many of them have been validated. There are also models of persistent forms of pain that are not related to an obvious injury but rather to a metabolic or hormonal dysfunction. These models attempt to study the functional pain condition with manipulations that don't involve actual injury or inflammation but that are related to the presumed cause of the pain, be that a hormonal imbalance, prolonged stress, or developmental alterations.

The current situation regarding the assessment of pain in animals can best be described as unsatisfactory. The models described in the preceding paragraphs are useful for studying some elementary mechanisms of injury detection but unlikely to give much information about more complex aspects of pain perception. Scientists are trying to develop new methods for the assessment of pain in animals, particularly of those forms of pain that are relevant to human pain and can be used to discover new pain treatments. Among the new paradigms and approaches being explored are the assessment of spontaneous pain and the detection of subtle reactions to discomfort (e.g., facial expressions or complex behavioral patterns that require a decision-making process indicative of the pleasant or unpleasant nature of the stimulus that caused it).

Studying basic mechanisms of injury detection helps to achieve deep insights into the molecular elements of the process. The pain sensor of a mouse or that of a snail uses molecular mediators for its activation that are the same across species, including humans. The most elementary the mechanism, the greater the chances of finding common pieces of machinery in many animal species. The problems begin when we want to assess the pain experiences of the animal, because the inter-species differences in pain perception are considerable. In addition, moving from a very basic molecular mechanisms involved in injury detection to a complex pain experience is problematic. The neurophysiologist Edgar Adrian, who in 1932 shared a Nobel Prize with Charles Sherrington for work on the functions of sensory neurons, made it very clear: "There may be many pitfalls in an argument which equates sensation in man with nervous discharges from the frog's skin."

Moving from molecular studies of injury detection to the assessment of pain in animals is the real challenge. Some scientists are calling from restricting the use of experimental animals to the study of very basic molecular processes, which can be done in isolated cells and tissue cultures, and using human volunteers or patients to study the more complex aspects of pain perception. Using modern non-invasive techniques of brain imaging coupled with verbal communication is a potential way forward. We will have to test new compounds on animals before they are used in humans, but the search for an ideal animal pain model that is both relevant to clinical pain and humane to the animals may be impracticable. Society is moving rapidly to giving animals greater protection by extending our own perceptions of pain to them and by eliminating unnecessary suffering. We probably will never know what the pain experience of a laboratory mouse is or how this experience conditions its behavior. Scientific assessment of pain in animals may be an attainable goal, but human nature will still compel us to give them the benefit of the doubt.

3 Nociceptors: Sensing Pain

When humans began making tools, one of their first priorities was the construction of weapons with which to inflict damage on their enemies. Soon they learned that injuries to the eye produced loss of vision and that damage to the ears led to deafness. By observing the consequences of injuries and diseases, mankind knew from the beginning of time that there was a close relationship between each sense organ and each sensation. Around 500 BC, a disciple of Pythagoras from southern Italy, Alcmaeon of Croton, studied the mechanisms of sensory perception. Having already decided that the brain was the seat of understanding, he wanted to know whether sensory perception required a direct connection between the brain and the sense organs. It is said that he tested this hypothesis by cutting the optic nerves of live animals and observing the ensuing loss of vision, which earned him the dubious distinction of being the inventor of vivisection. He concluded that all sense organs were connected to the brain by nerves, and that these connections were necessary for the perception of each individual sensation. His achievement was to synthesize these facts into a plausible explanation that linked each sense organ to a specific sensation by means of a neural connection between the sense organ and the brain.

This was the knowledge that provided the foundations for the Aristotelian five senses: eyes are for vision, ears are for hearing, and so on. The basic understanding was that there were a number of peripherally located sense organs, which were connected to the brain by sensory nerves, and that the messages that flowed through these channels eventually led to the various perceptions: vision, hearing, taste, smell, and touch. Interestingly, the sensation of touch was credited to the entire skin rather than to a distinct sense organ, as was the case with the other four senses. As was noted in a previous chapter, this school of thought attributed pain and pleasure to the mode of activation of the sense

organs rather than to having a separate sense organ for either of these two feelings.

The Aristotelian model of sensory perception prevailed for a very long time. The received knowledge was that pain was not a sense but the result of excessive or inappropriate stimulation of any of the other sense organs. Therefore there was no need to look for pain sensors in the body. The work of Descartes in the seventeenth century hinted at the possibility that some forms of pain, such as the acute pain of an injury, could be signaled by special sensors whose mission was to detect damage and to warn the brain that something should be done about it—for example, that a limb should be removed from a source of injury. From then on, scientists began exploring the possibility that such pain detectors could be real. They based a new theory of pain perception on the existence of specific injury detectors in the body that were connected to regions of the brain where pain sensations and the appropriate reactions to injury were generated. The debate between the two scientific approaches—Aristotelian and Cartesian—continued into our era, and only now are we beginning to understand how injury is detected and what role our sense organs play in the generation of pain sensations.

Do we have sensors in our bodies whose only mission is to detect and signal injury and whose activation leads to the sensation of pain?

A Very Specific Doctrine

If a tree falls in the forest and no one is around to hear it, does it still make a sound? Corny as this old question may be, I still use it as a starting point with my students when discussing the mechanisms of sensory perception, even though I always hear a few sighs of "Oh no, not that one again!" from some members of the audience. This question is very important to understanding one of the most significant developments in the scientific study of sensory perception: the pompously named Doctrine of Specific Nerve Energies, set forth in a textbook of physiology by the German physiologist Johannes Müller around 1835. Before the Doctrine of Specific Nerve Energies was proposed, it was generally accepted that the senses provide us with an accurate perception of the external world, so that what we see, hear, touch, or smell is the reality of the physical world that surrounds us. What Müller proposed is that we have a very limited perception of the outside world, and that what we see, hear, touch, or smell is only the portion of the outside world for

which we have a sense organ capable of detecting it. "Sensation," he wrote, "is not the conduction of a quality or state of external bodies to consciousness, but the conduction of a quality or state of our nerves to consciousness, excited by an external cause." There is a lot more in the world than what we can see, hear, or touch. There are also many forms of energy around us of which we are entirely unaware because we lack sensors for them.

Therefore, the answer, to the old question about the falling tree in the forest is that falling trees never "make a sound", whether or not there is someone around. The sound that we hear when a tree falls—or any sound that we can hear, for that matter—is a product of brain function that results from the detection of a very small part of the spectrum of air waves that the tree generates when it falls. Our hearing sensors detect waves in the range from about 20 cycles per second to 20,000 cycles per second. The portion of the spectrum of waves made by the falling tree that is within this range generates neural signals in our inner ears that are eventually perceived as a sound by the brain. But this sound is not a physical property of the falling tree. We learn throughout our lives to interpret these brain perceptions as the sounds made by various events: a tree falling, a car passing by, a bird singing, or a child crying. Animals, or younger or older humans, have different auditory spectra, and the sounds they perceive from the outside world are different from those of a normal adult. A whistle used to train dogs generates sounds in the range of 16,000–22,000 cycles per second that are perfectly audible for a dog but almost imperceptible for an adult human. You may think that a dog whistle doesn't make a sound; your dog, if he could, would argue that it does.

You may be surprised to know that ice isn't really cold. What we call cold is the consequence of our having temperature sensors in our skin that, when activated by the temperature of ice, generate a sensory perception in our brain that we interpret as cold. If we didn't have such temperature sensors, ice wouldn't feel cold. Likewise with warm, hot, touch, the color red, or any other kind of sensory perception. We walk every day through a world filled with a reality of which we perceive only a fraction. We are surrounded by electromagnetic waves from radios, cell phones, and television stations without having the slightest sensation that all these signals are there. Yet they are as real as the trees we see and the birds we hear. We have built machines—cell phones and TV receivers—that can pick up these signals because they have the appropriate sensors. We are insensitive to radiation waves that can kill us;

hence the need to wear artificial sensors and extra protection in radioactive installations. We can't perceive infrared light, but many snakes can; they hunt their prey by distinguishing differences in temperature between them and the surrounding objects. Bats fly around by detecting echoes with wavelengths well outside anything that we can perceive. Some animals can sense the planet's magnetic field and orient themselves by this signal rather than by vision or sound. Other animals are sensitive to electrical fields, yet we humans can't tell whether a wire is live unless we touch it—not the safest way of detecting an electrical current. The world looks very different to each animal species, and it all depends on the kind and range of sensors that each animal has. We perceive the external world through the windows of our senses, and what we perceive is only the fraction of the real world for which we have a sense organ. This is the essence of the Doctrine of Specific Nerve Energies, and this is why the question of whether a falling tree makes a sound if no one is around is still relevant.

A strict application of the Doctrine of Specific Nerve Energies generates a difficult question for the sense of touch and an even harder question for the sensations of pain: where are the sense organs for touch and pain? The other four main senses originate from well-identified organs in the eye, the ear, the nose, and the tongue where nerve cells translate light, sound, and chemicals into signals that generate images, sounds, tastes, and smells. However, in the case of the sensation of touch it wasn't easy to identify a unique sense organ as the source of the sensations, because the entire skin was supposed to be the organ of touch. It was therefore necessary to study whether such sense organs could be found in the skin and whether a correlation could be established between the individual components of tactile sensations (contact, temperature, texture) and the various kinds of sensory nerves that are found in the skin—and, along the way, to see whether the sensation of pain could also be attributed to a unique sensory organ in the skin, or to the pattern of stimulation of sensory nerves.

Detailed examination of the range of sensations evoked from the skin soon showed that the sensitivity of our external cover wasn't uniform. Some parts of the body are more sensitive than others to temperature, touch, or pain. The sensitivity of the skin is also not continuous; it is organized around sensitive spots surrounded by insensitive areas. Each spot corresponds to the place in the skin where we have a sensory nerve ending whose sensitivity determines the kind of sensation evoked from the spot. And so we have cold spots, warmth spots, touch spots, and pain

spots — a multitude of various kinds of spots surrounded by areas of skin devoid of sensitivity.

A natural consequence of the application of the Doctrine of Specific Nerve Energies to the sense of touch was a quest for an association between the elementary sensations evoked from the various spots and the kind of sensory nerve ending responsible for detecting and transmitting these signals to the brain. Many scientists participated in this search, and their names are attached to the various types of sensory organ found in the skin. Max von Frey, a German physiologist who worked at the turn of the nineteenth century, is credited with proposing a direct association between each sensation evoked from the skin and the nerve ending that detects those signals. He is also the inventor of the von Frey hair, a simple but clever device used to test for touch and pain sensations from the sensitive spots of the skin of humans and animals. The von Frey hair is still in use today in clinics and laboratories.

Von Frey set out to study differences in sensitivity between various regions of the body and to correlate those different sensations with the anatomical type of sense organ found in these locations. He tested himself, his assistants, and a large number of students and other volunteers. He tested all areas of the body including the cornea, the lips, the inside of the mouth, and even the tip of the penis, thus demonstrating that he saw no obstacles in his quest for knowledge. He concluded that the sensation of touch is mediated by the nerve endings that are associated with hair follicles in hairy skin and with a special kind of sensory ending known as Meissner's corpuscle in those areas of the skin that are devoid of hair. He also associated the sensation of cold with a nerve ending known as Krause's end-bulb and the sensation of warmth with a nerve ending called Ruffini's end-organ. This list of names and eponyms survived well into the 1960s. I still remember the aide-memoire that we used in medical school: "Krause the German is cold and Ruffini the Italian is warm." Von Frey's list of correlations also attributed the sensation of pain to the activation of nerve endings without a specific sense organ, which were called free nerve endings.

Von Frey's basic ideas were in line with the Doctrine of Specific Nerve Energies, and the concept of an association between each kind of sensory nerve ending and the sensation produced by its activation has survived the test of time. Unfortunately, von Frey got virtually all the associations wrong. His is a case of the right idea generating the wrong data, a familiar problem for many scientists. Today we know that all the corpuscles and end-organs named after the scientists that described them are, in fact,

involved in the detection of the mechanical properties of the objects that come into contact with our skins and therefore are involved, in one way or another, in tactile sensations. Some detect the actual contact and generate sensations of touch; others detect the velocity and acceleration of objects and are involved in the tactile recognition of objects' shapes and edges. We also know that sensory nerves without any specialized end-organ, the so-called free nerve endings, mediate the sensations of cold and warmth. The only association that von Frey got right was between pain and free nerve endings (and even that is not a unique association, as we have just seen with cold and warmth).

The most important idea to emerge from the Doctrine of Specific Nerve Energies was not that there should be an association between the anatomical appearance of a sense organ and the sensation evoked from it. We may be able to establish such correlations in some cases, but they aren't essential to understanding sensory perception. What it is important, though, is the idea that each sensor in our body detects a limited range of a particular kind of energy, and that this range determines what kind of sensations we can perceive. This range of a particular form of energy is known as the *adequate stimulus* of a sensory nerve. The concept of adequate stimulus includes the kind of energy to which the sensor is sensitive and the range of that energy that it can encode. Various forms of energy can activate many of the sensors in our bodies, but there is only one for which the sensor is exquisitely sensitive: its adequate stimulus.

Consider, for example, the sensors in our retinas. The Doctrine of Specific Nerve Energies tells us that they are our windows to the world of light, and that no matter how they are activated they will generate perceptions associated with light. Their adequate stimuli are electromagnetic waves in the range between 380 and 750 nanometers, the portion of the spectrum that we call visible and which corresponds to the colors between violet and red. We can't see anything outside this spectrum, and we call the outside edges ultraviolet and infrared. Within the visible spectrum our brains give us wonderful perceptions of the outside world with colors that correspond to this wavelength spectrum. But our sensors in the retina can also be activated by inadequate stimuli (for instance, by the mechanical energy of a punch in the eye), and although the perception will also be visual it will only generate a brief flash of light. The perception will also be unrelated to the magnitude of the stimulus; a punch twice as hard will not necessary result in our seeing twice as many stars or a flash of light twice as bright. Stimulating our sensors adequately

allows the brain to generate a meaningful sensory perception; stimulating them inadequately will produce only a meaningless perception of the same modality. Our sensors have the property of selective excitability; they are very sensitive to their adequate stimulus and much less sensitive to other forms of activation.

In our search for a pain sensor, we must therefore ask the following questions: What is the adequate stimulus for pain? Can we find sensors in our bodies whose adequate stimulus is the same stimulus that produces pain? And—should we find these pain sensors—would their activation be necessary and sufficient to produce pain? To answer these questions we need to look at the ideas and observations that generated the notion most closely associated with a pain receptor: the notion of the nociceptor.

Are Nociceptors the Pain Sensors?

As was discussed in chapter 1, Charles Sherrington thought that the elementary unit of brain function was the reflex, a simple network of nerve cells that worked by extracting information from the environment and generating timely and appropriate responses to the changes detected. You burn a finger and your muscles move the hand away from the heat source. More elaborate responses are the results of more intricate reflexes that add complexity to the simple reflex. Eventually memory, learning, and other higher functions emerge from this progressively complex network of reflexes. An important element of the correct functioning of the network is the recording of very accurate information about what is going on in our environment. If we look at how the elementary reflex behaves when we stimulate the body, then we will be able to deduce what kind of sensors the system has. That was Sherrington's line of thought.

Sherrington noted that elementary reflexes could be triggered by various kinds of stimulation applied to the skin. Some of these stimuli were simple touches on the skin which, in the appropriate circumstances, could evoke a startle reflex; for example, you are walking down a dark alley late at night, something or someone touches you on one shoulder, and you jump. Therefore we must have sensors in our skin that are very sensitive to the slightest touch and are capable of driving the reflex network. Sherrington called these sensors tango-receptors, deriving that term from the Latin tangere, meaning "touch." Because of its close association with the famous Argentine dance, this word didn't become very

popular in sensory physiology, and it didn't stick. Today we call these receptors low-threshold mechanoreceptors. A longer name, less erudite but very accurate.

Sherrington noticed that many different stimuli, all of which were able to produce injury, could also trigger the simple reflex very effectively. He also noticed that the motor response was always the same whether he used temperature (high or low), mechanical stimulation, or chemical stimulation. The only property common to all these stimuli was the capacity to inflict injury and damage to the skin. Thinking that there must be sensors in the skin capable of responding to all these various forms of energy, Sherrington called these sensors noci-receptors, or nociceptors for short, meaning sensors of noxious (or nocuous, as Sherrington put it) events. Commenting on their sensitivity to an unusually wide range of different kinds of stimulation, he wrote: "Instead of but one kind of stimulus being their adequate excitant, they may be regarded as adapted to the whole group of excitants, a group of excitants which has in relation to the organism one feature common to all its components, namely, a nocuous character."

The idea of an injury detector or nociceptor was therefore born as a speculative concept based on the observation of reflex responses. But, at the same time, some fundamental ideas about pain perception were also put forward. I have already commented on the notion of nociception (the processing by the brain of injury-related information)—a concept that separated the perception of pain from the study of how the nervous system deals with responses to damage. Linked to both the idea of nociception and that of the nociceptor is the concept of noxious stimulus as the adequate stimulus for nociceptors and therefore as a potential source of pain. A noxious stimulus is qualified by its ability to produce injury, whether this is done by mechanical, thermal, or chemical energy. A noxious stimulus is the adequate stimulus for nociceptors.

Nociceptors are thus defined as sensors that respond to forms of energy that can produce damage and injury to our bodies. Because their adequate stimulus is not linked to the type of energy that activates them (as with the other sensors) but to the capacity of the stimulus to inflict damage, they can be sensitive to more than one form of energy. Nociceptors are injury detectors. We now know that nociceptors exist all over the skin, in most internal organs, in muscles and joints, and in all other parts of our bodies from which we can experience pain after injury. Nociceptors are not associated with complex sense organs, and anatomically they are the free nerve endings that von Frey first identified as the

pain sensors. These sensors are the endings of the thinnest of all nerve fibers: A-delta and C fibers, which are the nerve fibers with the slowest conduction velocity of their nerve impulses. It is somewhat paradoxical that nature decided to use the slowest nerve pathways to transmit the signals that warn us of injuries.

The properties of the adequate stimulus for nociceptors tell us what kind of stimulations will be perceived as painful. There are basically two kinds of nociceptors: those that respond only to high-intensity mechanical stimulation and those that respond to several forms of high-intensity stimulation, including low and high temperature, high-intensity mechanical energy, and pain-producing chemicals. The latter group of nociceptors are universally known as polymodal, an adjective coined in the 1960s without taking into account that the first rule of taxonomy is not to mix Greek with Latin. Purists would prefer multimodal, but such is life.

These properties also help to explain some interesting aspects of pain perception, especially of the pain produced by acute injury. Polymodal nociceptors respond equally to skin temperatures greater than 45°C and lower than 20°C, which explains why we perceive both extreme heat and extreme cold as the same burning sensation. As we will see in the next section, all forms of energy that activate polymodal nociceptors, including chemical stimulation, generate a similar and intense burning feeling. This is a consequence of the fact that sensory perception depends on the type of sensor that is activated by the stimulus and not on the form of energy that activated it. Remember the point about seeing flashes of light when you get punched in the eye. On the other hand, noxious stimuli that can't activate nociceptors are essentially painless even if they produce injury. For instance, nociceptors can't be activated by radiation, and therefore we are insensitive to this form of energy. Some noxious stimuli are indeed adequate stimuli for nociceptors, but nociceptors can't detect all kinds of noxious stimuli. And the stimuli they can't detect are painless regardless of their ability to provoke injury.

In the last 40 years, nociceptors have been identified in all tissues of the body, and their responses to injury have been studied in great detail. These studies have reinforced the opinion that they are indeed the sensors that signal injury and that they are concerned with the generation of pain sensations. But some doubts remain as to what is the precise relationship between the activation of nociceptors and pain perception. Is the activation of a nociceptor sufficient to produce pain? Is pain a necessary consequence of the activation of nociceptors?

The first question has been partially answered with the use of micro-neurography, a technique that involves the recording of the electrical impulses generated by individual sensory nerve fibers in a conscious human and the subjective report of the sensations perceived by the subject when these fibers are stimulated. Thanks to microneurography we know the elementary sensations of touch evoked by the stimulation of different types of tactile sensory nerve fibers. But when it comes to pain and nociceptors there are some problems. First, this technique is mainly applied to superficial nerves, and to this day we don't have a subjective report of the sensations evoked by the stimulation of identi-fied nociceptors from internal organs. And even in the case of skin nociceptors it isn't easy, or even possible, to restrict the micrographic stimulation to a single fiber connected to a uniquely identified nocicep-tor. We know that stimulation of single tactile fibers, which is indeed possible, doesn't generate sensations other than touch in normal skin, but we still don't have unequivocal evidence that activation of a single noci-ceptor always evokes a pain sensation. We also know that under certain conditions—for example, when prolonged but not very intense heat is applied to the skin—nociceptors can be activated without this stimulus generating a pain sensation. Activation of nociceptors can indeed evoke pain, but we need an intense stimulation and a summation process to evoke a sensation of pain.

Trying to answer the second question has revealed an important caveat as to the role of nociceptors in the perception of some forms of persistent pain. The responses of nociceptors to noxious stimuli correlate well with the pain of acute forms of injury but don't explain satisfactorily chronic forms of pain in which the relationship between injury and pain is lost. We know that under certain circumstances pain can be evoked by activa-tion of tactile sensors of the type that normally evoke sensations of touch. This touch-evoked pain is a common feature of many forms of chronic neuropathic pain. Also, there are some diseases that cause pain by an abnormal sensitivity of neurons in the brain and spinal cord without a clear relationship with the activation of peripheral sensors (nociceptors or otherwise). As we will see in the following chapters, there is a lot more to chronic pain and to the pain of disease than a simple chain of events triggered by activity in nociceptors.

It is nevertheless true that the generation of acute pain states begins with the stimulation of nociceptors in the skin, in muscles, in joints, or in internal organs. This is the type of nociceptive pain induced by trauma, surgery, or acute injury. It is always a consequence of intense activation

of nociceptors. How these sensors respond to the stimuli that trigger them and how their responses change after an injury and during an inflammatory process are important aspects of the function of nociceptors and of their role in the signaling of injury and inflammation.

Red-Hot Chili Peppers

A Mexican friend of mine always carries with him a bottle of the hottest Tabasco sauce (the habanero variety) when he goes out to have dinner. He claims that if he doesn't add this sauce to his food it will taste of nothing. For some of us, the tiniest drop of this sauce will set our mouths on fire and will prevent us from tasting anything, speaking, or even breathing. How can this be? The answer is capsaicin, a chemical contained in the hot peppers used in Tabasco and other such sauces and that is responsible for making them hot. Capsaicin is also used in spray form for personal defense and riot control, as it disables people who come into contact with it. It is also added to birdseed to prevent squirrels and other unwanted guests from eating it. How is it that birds can eat capsaicin without any consequences but squirrels and humans can't?

The first thing to take into account is that capsaicin is a natural product, present in various amounts in plants such as peppers. There is a scale—the Scoville scale—that classifies different hot peppers depending on how much capsaicin they contain. For example, a habanero pepper is nearly 200 times as pungent as a jalapeño. Capsaicin excites polymodal nociceptors, and by doing so it produces a strong burning sensation. Of course, nothing is burning in your mouth when you eat a hot pepper; you feel the burning sensation because your polymodal nociceptors are being stimulated even though no injury or burn of any kind is produced. And when polymodal nociceptors are excited the result is a burning sensation regardless of how they were stimulated. This is another example of the adequate stimulus and the Doctrine of Specific Nerve Energies.

Capsaicin works by binding to a molecule present in polymodal nociceptors known as the TRPV1 receptor, a member of a large family of TRP molecules involved in sensory signaling. This is a channel in the membrane of the nociceptor that, when opened by capsaicin, activates the sensor that sends nerve impulses to the brain. The result is an intense burning sensation, the same feeling as if the nociceptor had been activated by any other means. The difference in this case is that the sensation is not triggered by a burn or an injury but by the chemical activation of the nociceptor. Birds' lack of sensitivity to capsaicin is yet another

example of the relationship between activity in nociceptors and pain sensation. Because their nociceptors lack capsaicin-sensitive TRPV1 receptors, birds can't sense the pungency of hot peppers. This evolutionary oddity is conveniently exploited by peppers that use the gastrointestinal tracts of birds to spread their seeds around.

Another important aspect of the actions of capsaicin is that prolonged exposure of nociceptors to this chemical renders them insensitive to it, a process known as desensitization. Moreover, if nociceptors are strongly activated by capsaicin when they are still immature, perhaps shortly after birth, they are destroyed—a feature that has been used in laboratories to produce animals with reduced numbers of polymodal nociceptors. Desensitization is what happens to people who ingest large quantities of capsaicin early in life—eventually they become so insensitive to it that only large doses of the strongest hot pepper sauce will make them taste any flavor of the food they eat. Desensitization has been used in treatment of diseases characterized by enhanced nociceptor activity. Capsaicin-containing creams have been developed for the purpose of rendering nociceptors inactive after repeated topical application to the skin. Such creams are used for the treatment of joint and muscle pain associated with strains or backaches or in cases of peripheral neuropathy, such as that induced by diabetes. They vary in effectiveness, mainly because the initial activation of nociceptors that precedes their desensitization causes pain.

Perhaps the most interesting aspect of the capsaicin story is the link between the chemical sensitivity of the nociceptors, their sensitivity to hot temperatures, and the burning sensation associated with either form of nociceptor activation. When nociceptors were first studied experimentally in laboratory animals, the most convenient way to activate them was by the application of heat. They showed robust and reliable responses to high temperatures—a form of stimulation that was easy to produce and quantify in a laboratory, either by contact or by radiant heat. Polymodal nociceptors were thus characterized as heat sensors, and, since the sensation evoked by hot temperatures was that of burning, they were labeled as the mediators of heat pain.

However, it was soon discovered that nociceptors were truly polymodal and could be activated not only by heat but also by mechanical stimuli and by many chemicals, of which capsaicin was one of the most potent. Other chemicals contained in plants (the mustard plant, for example) were also stimulants of nociceptors, as were some painful animal venoms of spiders and insects. This chemical sensitivity also

extends to other skin sensors beyond nociceptors, especially those that signal temperature. Warm and cold receptors can be activated by naturally occurring products of plants and animals. One of the best-known products that do this is menthol, a constituent of mint plants. Menthol is a strong stimulant of cold receptors—a property that manufacturers of toothpaste, chewing gum, and breath mints use to make you believe that your mouth is refreshingly cold when all that really happens is that your cold receptors are chemically activated by the menthol in their products. Interestingly, TRPM8—the molecule to which menthol binds in cold receptors and the molecule that is responsible for their activation—is also a member of the TRP receptor family.

The chemical sensitivity of polymodal nociceptors extends well beyond the natural products of some plants or animals. They are also sensitive to chemical changes in their environment—especially to products of cell destruction, to chemicals released by injured cells, and to many of the substances generated during an inflammatory process, including the acidification caused by tissue damage. All these chemical stimuli, whether natural products of plants and animals or the consequences of injury and inflammation, evoke pain. In many respects, polymodal nociceptors could be more accurately labeled as sensors of pain-producing chemicals than as heat detectors. Evolution has given many plants and animals chemical weapons with which to keep their predators at bay. It has also given sensors to the predators to warn them of such dangers. And the sensation produced by these chemical weapons is an unpleasant feeling of pain that we label "burning" because it is also produced occasionally when these sensors are activated by heat.

If we think in terms of our natural habitat, it seems more sensible to develop detectors of danger from our daily encounters with aggressive plants and animals than to develop sensors of high temperatures that rarely occur. We are supposed to go around naked in a temperate climate—an excellent way of getting scratches from plants, bites from insects and other such creatures, and minor wounds from our daily activities. Having sensors that teach us through pain to avoid these encounters and that help us to heal from our daily scrapes is extremely useful. That these sensors have an additional sensitivity to very high and very low temperatures is even more useful. Chili peppers and other such plants have developed a smart way to protect themselves from hungry predators by producing the very chemical that binds to the molecule that activates pain sensors in the animals that eat them. Unfortunately, they couldn't predict that humans would be capable of transforming this

clever defense mechanism into an enjoyable (for some) gastronomic experience.

The Dynamics of the Pain Sensors

Winters in Canada are cold and very long. We go through weeks of ice and snow yearning for a Caribbean beach. Some people are so desperate that they can't resist the temptation to enjoy the hot sun immediately after they arrive at a sunny destination. And they pay for it. After a couple of hours soaking in sunrays, the skin turns bright red and the pain of sunburn arrives. The red skin and the intense pain will last for a few days, during which the slightest contact, even the weight of a thin shirt, hurts. Let us look at what happens.

It all begins with yet another consequence of the Doctrine of Specific Nerve Energies. The stimulus that will burn the skin is the ultraviolet component of sunlight, a form of energy for which we have no sensors. We feel the heat of the sun through our warm receptors and the intense light through our eyes, but we aren't aware of the ultraviolet radiation that is damaging the cells in our skin and triggering an inflammatory response. Only when the inflammation is well under way do we begin to feel its consequences, still ignorant of the stimulus that caused it. The body tries to help by darkening the skin with melanin, a pigment that absorbs ultraviolet radiation and generates the much-desired suntan. But it cannot do that quickly enough to counteract the effects of sudden and intense exposure to the sun. We are injured without pain because we lack sensors for the energy that causes the damage.

The pain is caused by the products of cell destruction and by the local inflammation of the skin produced by the ultraviolet light. Damaged cells release chemicals that activate skin nociceptors causing a spontaneous burning sensation localized to the zones that received the ultraviolet light. The inflammation of the skin also causes a vasodilatation that leaks plasma from the capillaries, releasing even more compounds that activate nociceptors. In the area of burned skin, nociceptors are being continuously and intensely excited, not by the stimulus that caused the injury, but by the skin's response to the injury and by the products released by the damaged cells.

And that is not all. The chemicals that excite nociceptors also change some of their properties, most notably their threshold for excitation and their level of excitability. As nociceptors are continuously excited, they generate greater and greater responses, and they begin to respond to the

slightest of stimuli—stimuli well below their normal response threshold. This property, known as sensitization, is unique to nociceptors; no other sensor in the skin shows such amplification. The consequence of the sensitization of nociceptors is that stimuli that were previously below the pain threshold now become very painful. Not only do you feel an almost constant pain as a consequence of the continuous activation of nociceptors; in addition, your sensitized nociceptors are now activated by light tactile stimuli.

The chemicals released by damaged and inflamed tissues sensitize nociceptors, lowering their response thresholds and increasing their excitability. This is a consequence not only of sunburn but of every form of injury and inflammation of the skin, the muscles, the joints, or the internal organs. Nociceptor sensitization causes spontaneous pain, enhanced pain sensitivity, and pain produced by stimuli that normally don't hurt. From a sensory point of view, the entire process is known as hyperalgesia, meaning increased pain sensitivity. Because this increased sensitivity occurs at the point of injury, we call it primary hyperalgesia. We also have a word to describe feeling pain by innocuous stimuli: *allodynia*, a word invented in the late 1970s and derived from the Greek words for pain and other, meaning pain produced by stimuli other than those that normally cause it. Allodynia produced by tactile stimuli is also referred to as touch-evoked pain.

Nociceptor sensitization is therefore responsible for primary hyperalgesia. We burn a finger and for a few days we feel spontaneous pain due to the hyperactive sensitized nociceptors. We also feel pain if we touch the burn—a form of allodynia caused by the enhanced sensitivity of nociceptors that now respond to very mild stimuli. The entire process is caused by the actions of chemicals released by the damaged cells and by a local inflammatory process that sensitizes nociceptors to further stimuli. Primary hyperalgesia ends when a wound is repaired and the local tissues get back to normal, moping up the chemicals that cause the nociceptors' sensitization. Hyperalgesia protects the wound from further stimuli and help us to heal. We know a fair amount about the cellular process of nociceptor sensitization, and we have identified many of the molecules that mediate this event. These molecules are targets for the development of anti-inflammatory and analgesic drugs that can act at a site of injury; such drugs are very useful for treating acute pain and for treating diseases characterized primarily by nociceptor sensitization.

Another characteristic aspect of sunburn, and of every other form of injury or tissue damage, is the redness that accompanies it. From the

moment when nociceptors are activated or an inflammation sets in, the skin becomes red, and it remains so for the duration of the process. This is known as flare. It is due to local vasodilatation that causes plasma to leak out of capillaries; the plasma leakage leads to the characteristic swelling of an inflamed area. This vasodilatation also occurs in non-visible parts of the body, including muscles, joints, and internal organs, leading to an increase in the flow of blood to the damaged area.

It has been known for some time that nociceptors play an important role in the generation of flare. The activation of a nociceptor also induces the release of chemicals contained within it that have powerful vasodilatation activity and that contribute to enhancement of the inflammatory process. Therefore, not only do nociceptors transmit injury-related signals to the brain, leading to pain perception; they also contribute to the generation of local inflammation at the site of injury, which in turn helps to accelerate the healing process. The local inflammation induced by the release of vasoactive compounds by the nociceptors is known as neurogenic inflammation. The mechanism is also labeled as an axon reflex, meaning that a motor action (the inflammation) has been triggered by a single neuron: the nociceptor. This is a rather unfortunate term, as it gives the feeling that a reflex is involved when in fact all that happens is that the same neuron, the nociceptor, can produce both sensory and motor actions. Thus nociceptors have the dual role of sensing an injury and being part of the solution to it. They warn the brain that damage has occurred; at the same time, they release the compounds that start the repair of the tissue at the site of injury.

One interesting aspect of nociceptor sensitization is well documented. It turns out that most tissues of the body have nociceptors whose threshold for activation is so high that they are activated only rarely. However, like any other nociceptor, they can be sensitized—but only after intense stimuli of the type that generates a substantial inflammation are applied. These nociceptors appear to be dormant, hidden in the tissue and not doing much until an inflammatory process sets. Not surprisingly these nociceptors were initially called sleeping nociceptors. Today they are referred to as silent nociceptors. They seem to be sensors of large injuries and of well-developed inflammations rather than quick and ready alarm sensors that warn us of impending or potential damage. Their responses to noxious stimuli are similar to those of ordinary nociceptors, though with a much higher threshold, and their sensitization process is also similar. Awakening of sleeping nociceptors is thought to be the cause of some forms of persistent pain. Their lack of responsiveness

under normal conditions and their sensitization by intense inflammatory stimuli suggest that they play a major role in the signaling of chronic inflammatory pain.

Pain, Pleasure, and Itch

More than 100 years ago an association was established between pain perception and the signals conducted by the slowest sensory nerve fibers, known as C-fibers. This generated a kind of scientific knee-jerk reflex that equated activity in sensory C-fibers with pain, a notion that appears often in the scientific literature on pain mechanisms. It is indeed true that many nociceptors—though not all—are connected with C-fibers, but the converse is not true. Some sensory C-fibers transmit information about other sensory modalities that, although directly or indirectly related to pain, are quite distinct both in terms of the nature of the sensation and in terms of the mechanisms involved.

I have already commented on the fact that the sensors of moderate warmth and cold are also connected with slow-conducting sensory fibers, including C-fibers. There is also a mechanistic connection between the process of injury detection and the mechanisms that signal warmth and cold: they involve closely related molecular components, and they often share the same neurons in the brain. Many chronic pain diseases are characterized by dysfunctions of temperature perception, or by pain sensations triggered or modulated by innocuous cold and other temperature changes. However, the sensory consequences of pain's being so closely associated with the perception of temperature remain a mystery.

Some sensory C-fibers appear to be involved in the perception of pleasurable sensations. The search for injury detectors resulted in the discovery of a population of sensory C-fibers whose adequate stimulus was a low-intensity, slow-moving mechanical stroke of the skin—a caress. It didn't escape the attention of the scientists that humans find such stimuli pleasurable and that many animals bond by a grooming behavior that involves light stroking of the skin. It is thought that these "cuddle sensors" are part of our brain mechanisms for pleasure, and it is remarkable that they seem to use the same kind of sensory nerve fiber as pain. Pleasure and pain have been identified since the times of Aristotle as the two opposite emotional drives of our behavior. It is an odd feature of human curiosity that, whereas the mechanisms of pain have been subjects of intense scientific inquiry throughout history, comparatively little is known about how pleasure is detected and processed by the brain.

Nevertheless, the little we know about the detection of pleasurable sensations implicates sensors connected with a nerve pathway similar to the one used by pain. This may be how the brain areas that process our emotions and that receive both signals weigh one against the other to elaborate an appropriate behavioral pattern.

Another sensation closely related to pain and mediated by sensory C-fibers is itch. Max von Frey classified itch as a weak form of pain, which handily eliminated the need to look for specific itch sensors. Itch is a very unpleasant sensation; however, we respond to it not by withdrawing from the stimulus, as is the case with pain, but with a compulsion to concentrate on the stimulus and scratch. For a few moments, scratching evokes a pleasurable relief, even though it makes the itch worse and tells you that in the long term this isn't really the solution to your problem. Pain is indeed one of the best ways to relieve itch, and there are some itch-relieving machines in the market that are based on the stimulation of nociceptors and the generation of unpleasant sensations that in turn relieve itch.

There is still much debate as to whether itch is a separate sensation from pain, mediated by its own sensors and having a separate brain pathway, or just another form of pain that uses the same sensors and brain mechanisms with a different form of activation. Itch is best produced by chemicals (e.g. histamine) that are released during an allergic process, but it is also produced by other products of cell damage, or even by natural products of plants (e.g. cowhage) that cause itch by a mechanism not related to allergy or to histamine. Itch also is caused by some diseases of the skin, and by certain compounds (among them opiates and bile salts). The pleasurable (and brief) relief of itch by scratching is one of the best examples of the contrasts and associations of pleasure and pain and shows how closely these two strong behavioral drives are related.

The Enchanted Loom: Pain Networks

We often read in newspapers and popular books that the human brain is like a sophisticated computer. That figure of speech has been with us since computers became commonplace. Before then, the brain was compared to a telephone switchboard, and earlier to an elaborate clock, an intricate optical device, or a convoluted hydraulic system of pipes. The brain has always been a source of wonder. Ever since it was acknowledged to be the seat of our thoughts and our emotions, we have compared its workings to the most complex kind of technology available at the time. We started a long time ago with a model of the nervous system based on fluids running through tiny pipes; we have ended up comparing the brain to a computer more powerful that any we can build.

The brain is, of course, neither a hydraulic machine nor a computer, though some of its properties resemble those of such machines. The truth is that we really don't know how the brain works. We have a few ideas, but we are still far from understanding the fundamental basis of its mechanisms. And so we attribute to our brains the properties of the most sophisticated technologies of our times, especially those related to communication and control. The analogy is not about the actual mechanism but about what the machine does and its level of complexity. Not many people know how a computer works, anyway.

The most significant breakthrough in our understanding of the workings of the brain occurred around the end of the nineteenth century, when, thanks to good microscopes and refined methods of staining biological tissues, scientists learned that we are made up of cells. The Spanish histologist Santiago Ramón y Cajal extended this cellular interpretation to the nervous system and proposed that all the workings of the brain were built around the connections that individual nerve cells make with one another. Two new words entered the scientific literature: *neurons* for the nerve cells and *synapses* for the contacts made between neurons.

Synapses were not seen as fusions of neurons but only as contacts that left a space between two adjacent neurons. Chemical messengers or *neurotransmitters* mediated the communication between neurons by being released by one neuron's synapses to act on the neuron that received the message. We know that this interpretation is basically correct because if we physically cut certain connections between neurons or interfere chemically with the work of the neurotransmitters we can modify or even eliminate basic functions of the brain, including sensations, emotions, and cognition. This interpretation of the workings of the brain has given us, ever since, a relatively simple blueprint for a system of information and control.

We see the brain as a network of individual neurons that send messages to one another through chemical messengers released at their synaptic points of contact. At any moment, our brain is engaged in millions of such interactions, which produce a network of communication that somehow (we aren't quite sure how) governs our movements, feelings, emotions, and thoughts. Charles Sherrington provided the most poetic vision of this neuronal network when describing the cerebral cortex as it comes to life after sleep: "The brain is waking and with it the mind is returning. It is as if the Milky Way entered upon some cosmic dance. Swiftly the head mass becomes an enchanted loom where millions of flashing shuttles weave a dissolving pattern, always a meaningful pattern though never an abiding one; a shifting harmony of subpatterns." It is said that Sherrington was referring to the programmed loom controlled by punched cards that was a marvel of mechanical engineering and an important element of the English industrial revolution—yet another example of a metaphor for the workings of the brain based on contemporary sophisticated technology.

Can we identify networks of neurons involved in the signaling and perception of pain? Is there such a thing as a pain pathway in the brain, a sort of highway for pain signals? How does the enchanted loom deal with the information that will eventually generate the perception of pain?

We already know that the brain tissue is made of individual cells (neurons). Though these neurons can have many shapes and sizes, each of them has a cell body that contains the nucleus, with its genetic material and metabolic machinery, and extensions or branches that are called *dendrites* (Greek for *trees*) because they look like the branches of a tree. One of these extensions is bigger and usually longer than the rest, sometimes a lot longer; it is called the *axon* (short for *axis of the neuron*).

Neurons make contact with each other when the ends of their axons reach the dendrites and cell bodies of another neuron. There are some variations to this basic rule, but let us consider this simple arrangement as an easy way of making a neuronal network.

The contacts made by the ends of an axon with the dendrites or cell bodies of other neurons are the synapses. These contacts occur by proximity, not by fusion, leaving a tiny gap—the *synaptic cleft*—between the two neurons. One of the most useful properties of synapses for making networks is that the exchange of information between the two neurons that make the synapse can go only one way: from the axon of one neuron to the dendrites and cell body of the next. This is so because communication through a synapse involves a chemical messenger, the *neurotransmitter*, that is released into the synaptic cleft by the terminals of the axon and acts on receptive molecules, known as *receptors*, located in the membrane of the dendrites and cell body of the next neuron. There is no similar arrangement the other way round. Synapses are therefore one-way valves that allow transmission of information from the axon of one neuron to the dendrites and cell body of the next. Ramón y Cajal defined this property in 1891 as the *law of the dynamic polarization of the neuron*, revealing a literary taste characteristic of his time and background. Regardless of the name, these are the bases of our understanding of how neurons communicate with one another, a way of thinking that has been with us for more than 100 years.

Another essential property of synapses is that the action of the neurotransmitter on the receiving neuron can be either excitation or inhibition, depending on the type of receptor that binds to the transmitter. The same neurotransmitter can excite the next neuron in some synapses and inhibit neurons in other synapses. In this way neuronal networks can transmit some messages and interrupt others. The fact that synapses can be either excitatory or inhibitory is another important feature of neuronal processing, as networks of neurons can be activated or deactivated depending on the properties of the receptor at the synaptic contact.

The next features of neuronal networks are those concerned with the connections that neurons establish with one another. Neurons receive synaptic contact from many other neurons carrying information from several potentially different sources. This is called *convergence* and is usually interpreted as a way for a neuron to know what is going on in several other places. The downside is that receiving information from several different sources can mask the origin of the information carried

by the message. This is particularly relevant in pain networks, since many neurons receive information from nociceptors as well as from other types of sensors not concerned with the signaling of injury. Whether such neurons are members of a pain network will be discussed later in the chapter. The opposite of convergence is *divergence*, in which a single axon makes synaptic contact with many other neurons, some of them remote from the contacting neuron. This allows a neuronal network to send the same message to several areas of the brain so that the information can be used for many purposes at the same time: feelings, movements, emotions, or thoughts.

If we take into account the basic organization of a neuron, with information being collected by its dendrites and cell body and transmitted through its axon to the next cells, and if we understand that synapses are one-way valves of information, that they can be excitatory or inhibitory, and that neurons can receive convergent inputs from many sources and send divergent information to several targets, we are very well equipped to understand the nuances of neuronal networks.

When exploring the properties of a network, we must identify the origins and the nature of its inputs, the functional characteristics of its synaptic organization, the distribution of information throughout the various elements of the network, and the final destination of the message. The overall property of such a network is what Sherrington called *integration*—a very useful word that qualifies the functioning of a network at a particular time, be it through increased excitation or inhibition or through channeling of the output toward a specific task (be that sensory, motor, or related to a cognitive function). Neuronal networks are indeed the enchanted looms of our brains. Dissecting their components can give us insights into how a particular brain function takes shape.

Or so we believe. The organization of the nervous system isn't that simple. We have been working with these basic principles for more than a century, and, as we add more knowledge, some of our beliefs require revision or qualification. For example, synapses exhibit considerable plasticity, and their normal activity generates changes in their physiology that in turn determine the development and the overall connectivity of the entire network. Brain cells other than neurons also contribute to the processing of information. Cells that were previously thought to be supporters of metabolic activity, or scavengers of undesirable molecules such as *neuroglia* and *microglia*, are now considered to be active players in many processes, including pain. Depending on the condition of the

network at any moment, the same neurotransmitter can be either excitatory or inhibitory to the next neuron. And we don't understand at all how a pattern of activity in a particular network leads to an emotion, to a thought, or even to the unpleasantness of a pain perception. Undoubtedly "there are more things in heaven and earth than are dreamt of in our philosophy".

The Crossroads of Pain

You pull a string and it rings the bell that hangs at the other end. A telephone operator plugs a cable into the appropriate socket and the two people at the end of the connection can speak to one another on their telephones. You type a command on your computer's keyboard and the machine faithfully executes the order. We have an intuitive feeling that any action that involves communication is the result of a direct connection between the origin of the order and the executed effect. And we have extended this interpretation to the workings of the brain, assuming that each brain function is the result of neuronal activity in a specific area of the brain. The challenge is to find where these areas are and work out how the neurons are connected to one another and to their input and output sources.

Descartes thought the perception of pain was the product of pulling a string at the end of a nerve. He also proposed that the alarm bell rang in the pineal gland, which was thought to be the seat of the soul. The pineal gland is a very small bit of the brain located right in the center of it, between the two brain hemispheres. Descartes liked order and organization; hence his enthusiasm for a control center that was truly central. This obsession with identifying brain areas each in charge of a different function was taken to an extreme at the beginning of the nineteenth century by the German physician Franz Joseph Gall, inventor of the pseudo-science called *phrenology*. Gall believed that every brain function, and therefore every mental faculty, was restricted to a different area of the brain, and that the sizes of these areas were proportional to the influence of the corresponding mental faculty on the personality of the bearer. Gall went beyond reasonable interpretation when he suggested that examining the bumps on the skull of a person would reveal the size of the bit of the brain underneath each bump, thus allowing assessment of the psychological profile of the person. Porcelain busts with words such as *prudence*, *wit*, *benevolence*, and *courage* written on the head are an artistic and enduring legacy of this nonsense.

A few years after the birth of phrenology, the French neurologist Paul Broca added scientific support to the notion of brain localization. Broca studied the brains of patients who had suffered from aphasia (a complex language disorder) and identified an area on the frontal lobes of the brain as the region concerned with the processing of language. Linking a lesion in a small region of the brain with the expression of a complex neurological disease showed that even the highest functions of the brain could be mediated by discrete networks of neurons. Since the time of Broca, the prevailing interpretation of brain function has been that sensory inputs from various sources are integrated in neural networks whose activity leads to the appropriate response, and that the last step in the elaboration of this response occurs in a distinct area of the brain. And so this bit of the brain is for vision, this one for hearing, that one for memory, and that one for language. Modern brain imaging techniques have, to some extent, reinforced this view.

How about pain perception? Where are the pain networks, and how are the neurons that make up the networks connected to one another? What do we know about the brain cells that deal with pain-related information? We have an intuitive feeling that pain begins with an injury somewhere in the body and that this information is handled by a chain of neurons along the nervous system whose activity eventually leads to a pain perception. This is probably far too simple, but it is the universal model that has been used to identify how neurons respond when the body is injured.

As we saw in the previous chapter, injury is signaled in the tissues of the body by nociceptors—sensory receptors that send information to the brain about the nature of the injury. We also know that there are separate categories of sensors in the periphery, some detecting touch, some temperature, and some injury. When scientists tried to follow these lines of information into the brain, the very first thing they found was that most neurons that respond to the signals sent by nociceptors also respond to signals from other sensors including those that are activated by non-painful events. And here is a huge problem right at the beginning of our quest in search of pain networks in the brain: Why has nature taken so much care to develop highly sensitive and specific sensors to detect injury if this specificity is lost inside the brain at the earliest possible opportunity?

Let us look first at the areas of the nervous system where this information from our body tissues arrives. Nociceptors and other peripheral sensors are located at the very ends of our nerves (or the very beginning

if we take a more functional way of looking at things). The information picked up by nociceptors is sent almost unchanged through the nerves and into the nervous system. Signals from the head arrive, via the trigeminal nerve, at an area in the brain stem where these nerve fibers make synaptic contacts with brain neurons. Nociceptors from the rest of the body send their signals through various nerves in the limbs and the body that terminate in an orderly fashion along the spinal cord: those from the lower limbs in the lower part of the spinal cord, those from the thorax in the middle of the cord, and those from the upper limbs in the neck area of the spinal cord. The area of termination of these nerves is known as the *dorsal horn* of the spinal cord and is equivalent to the corresponding area of the trigeminal nerve in the brain stem. The dorsal horn and its trigeminal equivalent are the first relay areas of sensory messages coming from all over the body. This is where the first synapses are located, and therefore this is the earliest opportunity for integration of the pain message.

Many pain scientists believe that if we understand how pain signals are processed at the very first synaptic relay we will be well equipped to understand how other neurons farther up the network deal with these signals. This makes a lot of sense. After all, we know a fair amount about how nociceptors respond to injury, and knowing the properties of the input to a system gives us a good start. Thus, working out how pain signals are processed in the spinal cord should be relatively simple and should give us clues to the functioning of other pain networks. Unfortunately, the first relay of pain signals in the spinal cord has proved to be a lot more complicated than we first thought.

Mingling and Networking

To begin with, consider the anatomy of the spinal-cord relay. Most regions of the brain show amazing geometrical organization that is often related to how brain neurons operate. The cerebral cortex, for example, is made up of organized layers with distinct neuronal types and connections. The cortex of the cerebellum is a wonder of geometrical connectivity, with axons running in parallel lines through the dendritic trees of larger neurons in a beautifully organized arrangement. I could go on waxing lyrical about neuronal geometry in the hippocampus, the retina, or the olfactory bulb, but not about the connectivity of the dorsal horn. Ramón y Cajal, responsible for much of the unraveling of neuronal connectivity, referred to the dorsal horn as a *maremagnum*, a word commonly used in

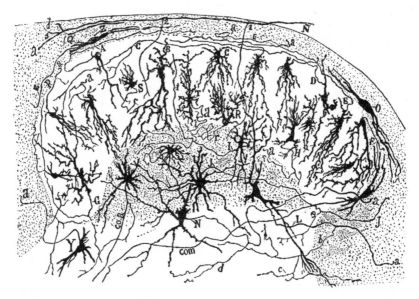

Figure 4.1
A drawing by the anatomist Ramón y Cajal of the neurons in the dorsal horn of the spinal cord, the first relay of sensory signals as they reach the central nervous system. Information from all kinds of sensors in the body converges on these spinal neurons with little selectivity. Ramón y Cajal referred to this part of the central nervous system as a maremagnum. This drawing was published in 1890.

Spanish to describe a confused and disorganized crowd of people and things (no direct English translation for this culturally-dependent concept). Ramón y Cajal called neurons in various other parts of the brain *climbing fibers*, *basket cells*, and *mossy fibers*, all expressions reminiscent of their beautiful connectivity. Labeling the dorsal horn a *maremagnum* was his admission of failure to find anatomical organization at the first synaptic relay.

Sensory nerves enter and terminate in the dorsal horn, making synaptic connections with second-order neurons without a clear pattern of organization. Detailed anatomical analysis of this region of the nervous system has shown that where there is some organization it is usually of sensory systems concerned with modalities other than pain. For instance, there is a very nicely organized set of contacts between the endings of sensory nerves that innervate hair follicles and the second-order neurons that transmit tactile information from the hairs to higher areas of the brain. The nerves that carry injury-related signals are the finest of all nerve fibers and terminate in the most superficial areas of the dorsal

horn. There they contact several types of neuron without any apparent pattern or specificity. Looking at the shape or size of a second-order neuron in the dorsal horn doesn't help us to discern what kind of sensory input it receives. Why the first synaptic relay of pain-related signals shows so little anatomical organization, whereas most other sensory modalities are well organized, is something of a mystery.

The spinal-cord endings of nociceptors connect with neurons in the most superficial layers of the dorsal horn, but some have also branches that reach deeper areas of the spinal cord. These very fine sensory fibers carry information from nociceptors but also from temperature sensors. As far as their areas of termination in the dorsal horn are concerned, they are indistinguishable from one another. Pain and temperature sensations seem to go together right from the beginning of brain processing, and they remain together for much of the journey along the brain—another puzzling fact. The areas of termination of sensory fibers in the dorsal horn are also dependent on the origin of the sensory receptor. For example, many nociceptors from the skin end in an area of the dorsal horn known as the *substantia gelatinosa* (meaning jelly-like matter), but those coming from internal organs, muscles, and joints seem to avoid that region. The substantia gelatinosa was thought to play an important role in pain processing because it received a large input from the finest-diameter sensory fibers, those involved in pain signaling. However, the fact that nociceptors from internal organs don't end in this area and yet pain from internal organs is as powerful as that from the skin calls into question the role of the substantia gelatinosa as an area uniquely concerned with pain processing.

When we look at the spinal-cord relay of the pain input from an anatomical point of view, there is little evidence of an ordered pattern of connections. There is some hint of organization in the fact that neurons in the superficial layers of the dorsal horn receive synaptic contacts from fine sensory fibers, mostly coming from nociceptors, but other than that the rest falls into the category of *maremagnum*. But perhaps this is the distinct aspect of pain processing: that a few neurons carry a restricted message about the source of the input and most other relay systems in the spinal cord are affected one way or another by injury-related information. Which component of this *maremagnum* is responsible for transmitting the information that will eventually lead to a pain perception is the crucial question.

The information we have on the functional properties of the spinal relay doesn't give immediate clues to the relevance of the various types

of dorsal-horn neurons to pain processing. Because of the very distinct groups of peripheral sensors, it would be expected that second-order neurons would retain this specificity. Yet one of the first things that scientists found when they explored the responses of dorsal-horn neurons to sensory inputs was that most of them responded to touch, to temperature, and to pain. However, more careful examination of the responses of spinal neurons demonstrated the existence of smaller groups of neurons with an exclusive response to a single sensory modality. Thus, two main types of dorsal-horn neurons have been identified: those that respond to many sensory inputs and those that respond only to one.

The first group is commonly known as *wide-dynamic-range* neurons— —a term lifted from the jargon of audiophiles in the mid 1960s, when these neurons were first described and when it was used in reference to audio amplifiers and tape recorders. These are neurons that respond to many types of sensory input, including touch, pressure, movement of hairs, temperature changes, and injury. Essentially they are activated by all forms of stimulation, innocuous or painful. They are also the largest group of dorsal-horn neurons, and for some time it was thought that they were the only kind that responded to injury-related signals. They are mostly large neurons located throughout the dorsal horn, and they tend to be connected with larger areas of the skin. They also receive sensory inputs from muscles, joints, and internal organs. Their range of responses is truly wide.

With time, other groups of spinal neuron were identified. Pain scientists were especially thrilled when neurons responding only to injury were first discovered. These neurons were called *nociceptor specific* because of their restricted input from nociceptors. They showed some special characteristics in addition to their limited range of responses. These neurons are located in the most superficial layers of the dorsal horn, where fine sensory fibers terminate, and are connected to smaller areas of the skin. Some also receive inputs from muscles and internal organs, and in these cases the inputs are also injury-related. They are good candidates for a dedicated network of pain-processing neurons but, alas, they are few in comparison with the much larger population of wide-dynamic-range (WDR) neurons.

The identification of these two classes of neuron at the very first synaptic relay of the pain network reopened the debate between specificity and pattern interpretations of how the brain deals with pain perception. The overwhelming evidence in favor of separate classes of sensory recep-

tors in the body—some responding to touch, some to temperature, and some to pain—seemed to support a strict specificity interpretation of pain mechanisms. Yet this specificity is seriously challenged at the very first opportunity for integration in the brain, at the spinal-cord relay. Moreover, as scientists explored other areas of the nervous system beyond the spinal cord they kept finding evidence that the most numerous type of neurons in the brain were those responding to a variety of inputs, innocuous and painful, and that those with a selective input from nociceptors were usually smaller populations of neurons restricted to certain regions of the brain. How can we interpret this mismatch between the high specificity of sensory inputs in the periphery of our bodies and the lack of specificity of many brain neurons?

There are several possible answers. One is that pain specificity is preserved in the nociceptor-specific population, a sensory channel that will accurately retain information about the painful nature of a stimulus. We only need a relatively small population of neurons to process this simple information, and therefore not a lot of them are engaged in this activity. The fact that the areas of skin from which nociceptor-specific neurons can be activated are small also suggests a greater role for these neurons in the discriminative aspects of pain perception. We could say that pain processing by the brain includes a direct line with selective information about the sensory component of the stimulus and a highly discriminative capacity.

On the other hand, an injury requires considerable processing of the motor, emotional, and cognitive reactions to it, from withdrawal of the body part to learning not to do whatever caused the injury again. Other, and larger, neuronal networks need to have injury-related information even if they aren't primarily concerned with telling the brain that an injury has occurred. The convergent properties of WDR neurons suggest that many of them may be involved in activities that require information as to whether there is also an injury somewhere else in the body. Convergence of pain inputs with other sensory modalities is a sign of modulation and plasticity and there is a lot of plasticity in the pain network. Neuronal inputs come and go as a result of persistent stimulation, prolonged pain, or even metabolic and hormonal influences. Having a population of neurons that are activated by several sensory inputs, including those related to injury, allows the brain to generate complex responses to a painful event. And this complexity requires many networks and many neurons; hence the larger number of WDR neurons at every relay point.

This kind of multi-sensory convergence isn't unique to the pain network. In the visual pathway, for instance, there are neurons that receive inputs from the retina and use that information to generate motor reactions, such as ducking to avoid an object thrown at you or grabbing that object. These neurons are part of the visual network but are not specifically concerned with the perception of an image. WDR neurons may be their pain counterparts.

There is, of course, another interpretation for the mismatch between the high specificity of sensory receptors and the convergence of inputs in the brain. It may be that the brain can extract a sensory message from the network's activity by means other than labeled lines or patterns of activity. To understand this we must look beyond this first relay in the spinal cord to see how pain messages are processed in higher centers of the brain. For many years scientists have been obsessed with the idea that the spinal-cord relay is a crucial area of pain modulation. General theories of pain perception were based on data from studies of the spinal relay, and this obsession limited their scope. Even today, pain perception is often equated with what happens at the spinal-cord relay. It isn't easy to explain this obsession with the spinal cord, and I am as guilty as anyone else having dedicated much of my research time to studying the spinal-cord mechanisms of pain. The combination of polarized opinions about specificity or pattern theories, messy anatomical and functional connectivity in the dorsal horn, and the lack of definitive data on the organization of the spinal-cord relay are responsible for this obsession. If we want to understand the more complex aspects of pain perception, we will have to look beyond the first relay. It is simplistic to think that pain perception will blindly follow the initial processing of the pain message at the spinal relay. A lot of mingling and networking precede conscious perception of a pain experience.

Via Dolorosa

Our understanding of the method the brain uses to deal with sensory perception is based on the existence of *sensory pathways*—highways for the transmission of information from the periphery of our bodies to a dedicated portion of the brain. This concept originates from the study of the senses (vision, hearing, smell, and taste) and from tracking of the neural connections from their respective sense organs (the eyes, ears, nose, and tongue) to the areas of the brain known to deal with the final perception of the sensory event.

These pathways were originally found by studying the consequences of brain injury. For example, damaging the occipital cortex (the portion of the cerebral cortex at the back of the head), or severing its connections to other brain areas or to the optic nerve, was known to render a person blind. Such observations helped to establish the origin and the termination of the visual pathway. Experimental surgery on animals added information about the details of the various pathways and gave support to the notions that for every sensation there is a sensory pathway from the peripheral organ to the brain and that along this pathway there are synaptic relays where the sensory message is modified until is transformed into a conscious perception in an area of the cerebral cortex.

No one questions that there are visual, auditory, olfactory, or taste pathways in the brain. Books and articles on the organization of these pathways are published all the time, and scientists talk openly about them. No objections are raised against naming any of these pathways for the sensations mediated by the information that flows through them. Yet for many years, standing up at a gathering of pain researchers and uttering the expression *pain pathway* would immediately trigger a barrage of condemnation, and the person in question would be reprimanded. The received knowledge was that there could not be such a thing as a pain pathway, because the injury-evoked signals transmitted through the brain couldn't be labeled with the word that qualifies a subjective sensation. As the signals travel through the brain, they aren't yet, and perhaps they never will be, the pain that is eventually perceived. Regardless of the fact that this argument would also condemn the use of expressions such as *visual pathway*, the intended effect was to reinforce the idea that pain is not a specific sensation mediated by a unique sense organ. In other words, Aristotle still rules.

In another chapter, I have discussed whether pain is a sensation similar to vision or hearing and the various views on the matter. Unfortunately, controversies over this question have influenced the analysis of the responses of neurons to painful stimuli and have made the study of a possible pain pathway very difficult. It is significant that pain researchers still argue about the use of expressions such as *pain pathway* yet scientists working in other fields of sensory neuroscience have no problem at all with visual or auditory pathways. And the greatest oddity is that the concept of a pain pathway and the data that supported its existence didn't come from scientists studying pain mechanisms but from surgeons and neurologists examining the consequences of lesions to various parts of the brain.

Physicians noticed that a lesion to the spinal cord that severed the antero-lateral region of the cord resulted in a loss of pain and temperature sensation from the opposite side of the body below the point of the lesion. Most of these injuries were traumatic, and the lesions weren't very restricted; however, it was always observed that if a patient had, say, a mid-thoracic spinal-cord injury that destroyed the antero-lateral region of the cord, no pain or temperature sensations could be generated from the abdomen and from the leg opposite to the side of the injury. This observation generated the idea of a pain and temperature pathway organized so that pain and temperature sensory fibers from the periphery make synaptic contacts with second-order neurons in the spinal cord whose axons then cross to the opposite side and ascend toward the brain in the antero-lateral region of the cord. This arrangement explained the clinical signs observed in patients with spinal-cord injuries and was consistent with what was known about the anatomy of the spinal cord. Animal studies provided experimental support, and the concept of a specific pain pathway running through the antero-lateral region of the spinal cord and into the brain was born. Interestingly, all these ideas made it into textbooks very soon after they were put forward and have remained there ever since.

The main consequence of the idea of a distinct and identifiable pain pathway was to give neurosurgeons an excuse to begin cutting bits of the spinal cord to treat severe pain. A procedure known as *antero-lateral cordotomy*, in which the antero-lateral region of the cord in the thorax or the neck was severed, was introduced to eliminate intense abdominal pain. In view of the irreversibility of the operation, the procedure was initially restricted to terminal patients with extensive abdominal cancer and the results were spectacularly good. Antero-lateral cordotomy produced a complete loss of pain and temperature sensations from below the point of surgery, and this made the life of those suffering from terminal cancer much more bearable. The success rate was so high that soon the surgery was also performed in patients with longer life expectancies to eliminate intense, untreatable, and persistent chronic pain. And then the problems began. Patients who died a few weeks or months after the surgery never recovered any sensation, but many of those who survived for longer periods of time eventually recovered some pain sensitivity. And the new sensitivity quickly developed into a pain equal to or even worse than the original one. The new sensations that appeared in the area rendered insensitive by the cordotomy were inconsistent, capricious, and not at all uniform from patient to patient. William Noordenbos, a

Dutch neurosurgeon who studied many cordotomy patients in the 1950s and the 1960s, concluded that the main problem with this form of surgical treatment of pain is that it was inconsistent and unpredictable.

If pain is transmitted by a spinal-cord highway of information from the periphery to the brain, then cutting this pathway should stop the pain forever. The facts that this doesn't happen in all patients, that some develop worse and weirder forms of pain, and that this new pain appears some time after the surgery tell us that there is a lot of plasticity in the nervous system and that pain-related signals can find alternative ways to reach their destination if the main road is closed. But they also tell us that there is indeed a pathway the mediates pain and temperature in the antero-lateral portion of the spinal cord, and that cutting it eliminates the pain in all people for some time and in some people forever. Thus, there is some truth in the concept of a pain pathway.

How is this *via dolorosa* organized? We know that the axons running in this pathway originate from neurons with cell bodies in the opposite side of the spinal cord; hence the crossed nature of the pain loss. These neurons receive inputs from pain and temperature sensors in the skin, the muscles, and the internal organs, and many of them also receive inputs from tactile organs. Not every signal in the pain pathway is related to injury. These axons terminate in various regions of the brain, where they make contact with other neurons that eventually carry the message all the way to the cerebral cortex. An important relay nucleus for the pain pathway is the thalamus, a big sensory nucleus in the middle of the brain; for this reason, the pain pathway is often identified with a spino-thalamic projection. But there are also other areas of termination of the spinal pathway, including regions of the brain that deal with hormonal controls, vegetative functions, and emotional reactions.

An interesting and somewhat mysterious aspect of the pain pathway in the spinal cord is that it transmits information related to pain and to temperature together. The pathway is still referred to in many textbooks as the *pain and temperature pathway*. Why do these two sensations travel together toward the brain? Some scientists think this has to do with the processing of the general feelings of the body (that is, with whether we feel good or bad) rather than with projecting a single sensation, but the fact is that we simply don't know why pain and temperature share the same pathway. We do know, however, that both sets of sensors are connected to the thinnest and slowest of nerve fibers in our peripheral nerves, and that they project together to the neurons that send messages to the brain through the antero-lateral portion of the spinal cord.

Thus, there is indeed a pain pathway running though the spinal cord, but cutting it doesn't guarantee that all such sensations will be interrupted forever. Maybe other pathways that also receive injury-related information can take over the traffic if this road is blocked. Perhaps new connections are made that bypass the obstacle created by the surgery. Clearly a spinal-cord pathway to the brain is not the whole story. There is a lot of plasticity in the connections that neurons establish with one another, and this plasticity offers alternative routes of information that the brain can use to generate pain-related signals. We need to see this system in action—that is, we need to study the dynamics of pain sensation and how pain can change so as to transform a painless event into a painful one.

5 Pain Dynamics: Sensitization

Think about the simple act of buying a new pair of shoes. You try them on in the shop, think they fit quite well, and walk a few steps to make sure they are reasonably comfortable. After that simple test, you decide to buy them. You know from experience that the first few times you wear them they are going to hurt a bit. If you are unlucky they may hurt a lot. A minor rub that in the shop was almost imperceptible may develop into an unpleasant pain. It may take a while for your feet to get used to the shoes. Only after they stop rubbing the annoying sore spots will the pain go away.

The problem with your new shoes is the consequence of a unique property of pain sensation: its inability to adapt. Every other sensory experience, after a prolonged and constant stimulus, adapts to a lower level or even stops being perceived altogether. If you walk into a room and there is an intense odor, it doesn't take long for you to stop perceiving the odor. You don't hear the rumbling sound of your washing machine after a few minutes. Interestingly, you can tell when the washing machine stops, because you detect that the noise has ended even though by then you weren't really hearing it. We have a powerful mechanism of *sensory adaptation* that eliminates a continuous noise or a persistent odor from our perceptual world and helps us to see in very bright or very dark conditions. Our senses are dampened by persistent and constant stimulation and are awakened by sudden changes and by contrasts. The alternating black and white stripes of pedestrian crossings and the two-tone sirens of fire engines and ambulances keep our senses alert to these important signals by preventing sensory adaptation. Nothing blunts our senses more than constant and uniform stimulation.

Pain is the only exception to the adaptation rule. In fact, pain not only doesn't adapt; it produces the opposite effect: it amplifies as it persists. Hence the problem with your new shoes. In the shop you may not even

have noticed the slight rubbing, and you would hardly have called it a pain sensation. Yet as this very small source of minor pain bombards your brain continuously, the tiny pain becomes progressively larger and larger. It amplifies to a point where wearing your new shoes may became torture. The amount of pain that you feel once the amplification process has set in is out of proportion to the minor rubbing. You are suffering the consequences of a process known as *sensitization*.

Using the tools of psychophysics (the science that studies the relationship between physical stimuli and the sensations they produce), sensory adaptation is revealed by a shift toward the right of the curve that relates stimulus intensity to sensory perception. This rightward shift means that after your senses adapt it will take a greater intensity of the stimulus to produce the same amount of sensation, and that your sensory threshold (the intensity at which you begin to perceive a stimulus) will be higher. However, when we use the same techniques to measure pain perception after a continuous painful stimulus, we note that the pain-perception curve has shifted in the opposite direction, toward the left, showing sensory amplification rather than sensory adaptation. Now, less intense stimuli produce more intense pain. We call this process *hyperalgesia*, meaning increased pain sensitivity. And because the pain threshold has also moved toward lower stimulus intensities, we may now feel pain at intensities of stimulation that hadn't been painful before. We have a special word—*allodynia*—for the feeling of pain caused by stimulations that don't normally produce pain. Allodynia and hyperalgesia are consequences of pain amplification, the properties that make pain unique among sensory perceptions and that demonstrate that pain doesn't adapt to prolonged and continuous stimulation.

The pain caused by your new pair of shoes is trivial when compared to the pain of patients who suffer from chronic pain. A pain that doesn't go away is a pain that increases and increases until eventually it dominates all aspects of a person's life. The lack of adaptation to pain is what drives many chronic-pain patients to anxiety and then to depression. The pain is always there. You may learn to live with it, but it will never go away. Pain amplification can be helpful under normal circumstances because it helps you to take care of an injured body part. This is essential for the healing process, and it is a consequence of the protective nature of pain. For people with chronic pain, however, the amplification of pain sensitivity expressed as allodynia and hyperalgesia becomes the dominant symptom of their diseases and ruins the quality of their lives. Pain amplification adds suffering to the unpleasantness of chronic pain.

Pain amplification is usually interpreted as a consequence of the sensitization of the neural mechanisms that normally mediate pain sensitivity. Whether sensitization is what causes the amplification of chronic pain or whether a persistent pain stimulus is what causes neuronal sensitization is a chicken-and-egg problem. The problem arises from the very use of the word *sensitization* and from its application to pain sensitivity and to the mechanisms that mediate pain perception. Thus, in order to understand the mechanisms of chronic pain we need to determine what sensitization is and how it contributes to the dynamics of pain sensitivity.

The Meaning of Sensitization

The word *sensitization* is used in many different contexts to mean many different things. It is used in several scientific disciplines, including immunology and neuroscience. It qualifies cellular and molecular processes, but it also describes behavioral patterns. Intuitively it suggests enhancement or amplification of a process. We can be sensitized to allergens or to politicians. We respond with a greater reaction, a lower threshold, or an increased annoyance to a persistent input.

The basic meaning of *sensitization* is of an increased reaction to a continuous and constant input. The reaction could be of a cell or of a whole animal, ranging from the enhanced excitability of a molecular process to an exaggerated behavioral reaction to an environmental stimulus. In connection with pain mechanisms, *sensitization* has been used in several contexts to describe the process of pain amplification, from the increased sensitivity of a single neuron to the enhanced pain perception of a chronic-pain patient. And this is precisely the problem. *Sensitization* has been defined and used in two completely different ways by different people seeking to qualify pain processes.

On the one hand, clinicians use *sensitization* as an all-encompassing term in regard to persistent pain. Patients with fibromyalgia, irritable bowel syndrome, or chronic osteoarthritis are said to suffer from conditions caused by sensitization of their nervous systems. The idea is that enhanced excitability of the parts of the brain concerned with pain perception leads to increased pain sensitivity. Unfortunately, these interpretations are hypothetical, as it is difficult to establish beyond reasonable doubt that any one of the chronic-pain states in question is caused by enhanced brain activity.

At the other end of the spectrum, *sensitization* is used by neuroscientists to describe a process of enhanced sensitivity of a single neuron or

of a group of neurons in response to continuous and persistent stimulation. In this case, *sensitization* refers to a precise and detailed cellular process whose relevance to a human sensory experience is hard to establish. Scientifically, sensitization in this second sense is the easier kind of sensitization to study, bearing in mind that we will have to guess what is the functional relevance of the process (if there is any). We can indeed record the activity of a single neuron in an area of the brain that we suspect has something to do with pain perception, and we can study the intricacies of the molecular process that generate its sensitization, but we can't simultaneously know what these signals mean for the overall perception of pain.

We pain scientists take a bottom-up approach to studying these pain dynamics. We look for processes that show changes in magnitude and temporal courses similar to those of the reported perceptions, and we hope that by progressively building up data and information we will one day achieve the goal of demonstrating that a certain molecular process is the cause of a certain chronic-pain condition. Clinicians work the other way round, starting with the complete repertoire of signs and symptoms of a chronic-pain patient and trying to tease out whether any of these symptoms could be due to one of several hypothetical mechanisms. Studying responses to a particular treatment helps them to see whether they are on the right track. The two approaches are complementary, and with time, effort, and a bit of luck we may eventually establish the connection between a cellular process and a clinical pain symptom.

As was noted in an earlier chapter, the word *sensitization* was first used in the study of pain mechanisms to describe the enhanced responses of nociceptors in peripheral tissues to repeated stimulation or to inflammatory mediators. These studies, begun more than 40 years ago, showed that the sensors in our tissues that signal injury—the nociceptors—lowered their response threshold and increased their excitability when subjected to repeated stimulation, to an injury, or to an inflammatory process. "Sensitization of peripheral nociceptors" was the expression used to describe this phenomenon, which was also thought to be responsible for the increased sensitivity to pain that occurs in peripheral tissues and organs after an injury or in the presence of an inflammatory process.

More recently, *sensitization* has also been used to describe the process of increased excitability of neurons in the spinal cord and the brain after a repetitive or persistent input from nociceptors. To distinguish this phenomenon from the one previously identified in peripheral tissues, it was further qualified as *central* sensitization. The study of central sensitiza-

tion opened new avenues for the identification of potential molecular mechanisms of chronic pain, which in turn generated many candidates for the title of "the pain molecule." Some of these candidates have been followed up by the pharmaceutical industry, with various degrees of success; so far, none of them has proved entirely satisfactory. Often the side effects of trying to block or modulate the actions of a certain molecule in the brain outweigh its possible analgesic benefits. In other cases, including that of the notorious molecular family known as *NK1-receptor-antagonists*, drugs that were shown to be highly effective in reducing central sensitization of pain pathways in experimental animals failed to demonstrate any analgesic effect when administered to patients.

The problem here is that sensitization of neurons after repeated stimulation is not unique or specific to pain processing. In many ways, this kind of neuronal sensitization is an intrinsic property of all synapses and a feature of the plasticity of neuronal networks. The molecular mediators of sensitization are present in areas of the brain concerned with cognition, memory, and learning, not just in areas concerned with pain. We could even say that the brain learns by a process of sensitization—the same process that the brain uses to amplify pain—and that this process can go wrong and can result in chronic pain. The challenge is to identify the molecular components of the sensitization process that are concerned with pain amplification and nothing else. That is the current goal of many pain scientists. Achieving it will be a decisive step in the discovery of useful therapeutic targets for the relief of chronic pain.

The Three Crucial Processes of Pain Dynamics

Pain is a dynamic and changing sensation that doesn't adapt to a constant stimulus and that increases as it persists. Under normal circumstances, pain amplification is an expression of the brain's ability to adapt to a hostile environment, a useful property that reminds us to shield our injuries and helps us to heal. But when pain doesn't go away after an injury has healed, or when there never was an injury in the first place, or when there is nothing to adapt to, the amplification of pain, which is intrinsic to its own mechanism, becomes not only useless but also a nuisance. From a mechanistic point of view, the processes that mediate pain amplification are always there, normal components of the biology of the brain. If expressed appropriately, in response to an injury, they are useful and protective. But if triggered by disease or by a maladaptive reaction to an external stimulus, they can result in chronic, pathological pain.

The three crucial processes that are believed to contribute to pain amplification are all expressions of neuronal sensitization, and their magnitude and time course match those of persistent pain. The evidence for their role in persistent pain is substantial and compelling, but they are also likely to contribute to reactions of the body to injury other than the perception of pain—for example, changes in cardiovascular control, in respiration or in motor activity. We are still not quite sure how much of the neuronal sensitization that we can detect in animal models contributes to pain perception in humans, or whether the enhanced neuronal excitability that characterizes sensitization is unique to the perception of pain and related to pain hypersensitivity.

The first crucial process is the sensitization of peripheral nociceptors. The sensors in our bodies that respond to injury can change their properties as a consequence of the very injuries that they detect. Products and mediators of tissue inflammation, substances released by the cells damaged by the injury, and transmitters secreted by the nerves of a damaged area can all contribute to changing the excitability of the nociceptors in the region of injury and making them more excitable. As a result of this process, nociceptors are transformed into sensors that respond to low-intensity stimuli and that are active even in the absence of a stimulus. The process of nociceptor sensitization is believed to be responsible for the increased pain sensitivity felt at a point of injury or associated with a localized inflammatory process. Nociceptor sensitization contributes to the spontaneous pain felt after an injury and to the pain evoked by low-intensity stimuli, such as touch or light contact, at the point of injury. It could also be that nociceptors are sensitized in the absence of a clear injury or an overt inflammatory process. In such cases, the sensitized nociceptors may mediate pain sensations from regions of the body that are apparently normal, a form of pain known as *functional* pain. There is a current of opinion among scientists and clinicians that the pain of irritable bowel syndrome or that of interstitial cystitis is caused by such a mechanism, although direct experimental proof is still lacking.

The second crucial process is the strengthening and reinforcement of synaptic transmission between neurons that mediate pain signals in the spinal cord and the brain. To differentiate this process of sensitization from the sensitization of nociceptors in peripheral tissues, it is called *central* sensitization. The idea is that the continuous arrival in the central nervous system of the signals sent by peripheral nociceptors from a region of injury strengthen the contacts between the neurons in the

spinal cord and the brain that are in charge of processing pain-related information. And in doing so the pain pathway becomes more excitable and more active and maintains its hyperactivity over and above the duration of the injury, which leads to persistent and enhanced pain. The process that mediates this function is the plasticity of the synaptic contacts between the neurons that don't behave in a fixed and rigid manner but are able to become more active and to increase their transmission capacity in the presence of a barrage of signals from a site of injury. Synaptic plasticity is at the root of central sensitization. As we will see later in the chapter, this is why pain hypersensitivity shares mechanistic features with other brain functions (such as memory) that depend on the plasticity of neuronal connections.

The third crucial process that contributes to pain hypersensitivity is the ability of information from touch sensors and other low-threshold receptors in peripheral tissues to activate pain-generating systems in the spinal cord and the brain, particularly during prolonged pain. This is a remarkable property of the pain system and a fascinating function of the brain. Under normal circumstances, the activation of nociceptors produces pain and the activation of touch sensors produces touch, as is logical and expected. But after an injury, as a result of an inflammatory process, or sometimes even in the absence of a peripheral injury, the activation of touch sensors gains access to the pain-processing channel of the brain and a tactile stimulus generates a pain sensation. This is an amazing transformation, as amazing as if suddenly a sound were to produce images in your brain or a picture were to generate sensations of smell or taste. For a long time it was thought that the phenomenon of touch-evoked pain that is characteristic of many chronic-pain states was mediated entirely by the sensitization of peripheral nociceptors—a logical interpretation. But now we know that what happens in many cases is that information from tactile sensors that normally are concerned with the generation of the sensation of touch gains access to the pain system and produces painful sensations, and thus pain is evoked by low-intensity contact and tactile stimuli applied to the skin.

A common feature of these three essential processes of pain hypersensitivity is the alteration of the input-output relationship that defines the kind of sensation produced by a certain incoming signal. Normally we expect a light contact tactile stimulus applied to our skins to produce the sensation of touch, and a brief or minor injury to produce a brief and minor pain sensation. But if we examine the consequences of the three processes just described, we notice that in each of them there is a

disproportion or even a complete mismatch between the input and the output. A sensitized nociceptor responds to low-intensity stimuli such as touch, a sensitized synapse will transmit a more intense message than the one it receives, and an altered tactile pathway that is now able to gain access to the pain system will transform a touch stimulus into a pain sensation. In each of these cases, the physical reality of the stimulus is transformed into a perception that differs from the physical reality in magnitude, in quality, or in both magnitude and quality.

One might think that a brain that generates perceptions that fail to match reality is not a very refined brain. On the contrary, this is the hallmark of a very sophisticated thinking machine. Your brain works, for pain perception and for everything else, by producing images and sensations that best help you to make correct decisions about every aspect of your life. Sometimes these images and perceptions are very precise, but often they are not at all direct reflections of the originating stimulus, and occasionally they are far from accurate.

Here is an example involving the visual system. Read the following sentence:

Aoccdrnig to rscheearch at an Canaidan uinervtisy, it deosn't mttaer in waht oredr the ltteers in a wrod are, olny taht the frist and lsat ltteres are at the rghit pcleas. The rset can be a toatl mses and you can sitll raed it wouthit a porbelm.

Your eyes have transmitted the letters faithfully to your brain in the order in which they are printed. But your brain has refused to accept this stimulus and has ordered the letters not as they are printed but in a way that helps you to understand the sentence. The final perception and the act of cognition that allows you to understand the sentence aren't direct transcripts of the stimulus presented.

There are many examples of such transformations, you can spend a few hours in the Internet enjoying them, but let's go back to pain perception and pain hypersensitivity. For many years scientists have wondered how is it that after injury or inflammation or in some pathological pain states there is so little correspondence between the nature of the stimulus and the kind and magnitude of the pain sensation. The simple answer is that this is how the brain *always* works. It works by transforming the external reality into perceptions that give meaning to your actions—a process that sometimes requires profound modification of the reality presented to us. If you need to protect an injured limb, to stop eating after a digestive insult, or to reduce your activity in order to nurse an

inflamed joint, your brain will transform every innocuous stimulus to your limb, your stomach, or your joint into an unpleasantly painful sensation. It is in your best interest in all these situations to feel pain when touch is applied, even if that means that your perception is very different from the reality of the stimulus. Pain hypersensitivity and the consequences of sensitization are, under normal circumstances, examples of the capacity of the brain to adapt to a changing and hostile world. And when something goes wrong and the brain malfunctions, as in the case of neuropathic pain, the abnormal pain sensations don't match the causing stimulus and may even appear in the absence of a stimulus. Dissociations between stimulus and perception are a feature of the normal workings of the brain and a potential source of pathology in abnormal pain states.

Amplifying Your Pain

If sensitization is a source of chronic pain, identifying molecules that cause the sensitization process may enable us to discover new therapeutic targets for pain relief. Before the present ideas about sensitization and pain amplification were developed, the search for analgesics was aimed at reducing or abolishing pain—all kinds of pain, including the good and protective and the useless and pathological. But if we now believe that the enhancement of pain sensitivity is what makes pain persistent and unpleasant, then reducing the sensitization process would restore pain to its normal levels and maintain the protective nature of an alarm system without the excesses of its amplification. The therapeutic quest changed from searching for *analgesics* (drugs that abolish pain) to searching for *anti-hyperalgesics* (drugs that reduce the enhanced sensitivity of the pain system without affecting the normal perception of pain). And when searching for anti-hyperalgesics, we need to know which cellular and molecular mechanisms mediate the three fundamental processes of pain sensitization.

Products of tissue injury and inflammation mediate nociceptor sensitization. The damage caused to a tissue by an injury releases many compounds that produce two separate effects: they trigger an inflammatory process aimed at healing the injury and they change the excitability of the nerve sensors in the injured tissue. Inflammatory mediators, of which there is a constellation commonly referred in the trade as the *inflammatory soup*, don't directly activate nociceptors, but contribute to the sensitization process and to the increased excitability of nociceptors that in

turn leads to enhanced pain perception from an injured region of the body. The sensitization process lasts as long as the inflammation, and if not resolved satisfactorily it can outlast the healing time and generate chronic inflammatory pain. Drugs aimed at reducing the inflammatory process associated with injury, from the humble aspirin to the more modern anti-inflammatory compounds, decrease pain by reducing tissue inflammation and hence reversing the sensitization of peripheral nociceptors.

We also know that tissue injury and inflammation trigger over-expression of the molecules responsible for controlling the excitability of nociceptors. The consequence is a set of more excitable sensors, with lower thresholds for activation, enhanced responsiveness to their normal stimuli, and spontaneous activity, all of which can generate increased and spontaneous pain. Among the molecules that can be over-expressed in nociceptors during injury and inflammation are the channels that control the flow of ions in and out of the nerves and that generate the nerve signals that are sent toward the brain. Some of these channels, especially some forms of sodium channels, are directly related to the sensitization process and have been identified as targets in the enhancement of excitability of tissue nociceptors that leads to pain hypersensitivity from an inflamed tissue. One such sodium channel, known as *Nav 1.7*, was recently identified as playing an important part in the generation of pain signals from peripheral tissues. Members of several Pakistani families were found to exhibit "congenital insensitivity"—a complete lack of pain sensitivity caused by a genetic loss of Nav 1.7 channels in their peripheral nociceptors. This and studies of other types of ion channel in nociceptors have generated much knowledge about the details of the process of nociceptor sensitization and opened new avenues for the development of drugs that have the potential to reduce or abolish the enhanced pain sensitivity associated with tissue injury and inflammation.

Research has also focused on the study of the mechanisms of pain sensitization in the spinal cord, where pain signals first enter the central nervous system. The rationale of these studies is that knowing how pain messages are modified at the first opportunity will give us clues to how these messages are handled throughout the brain. Numerous studies have looked for molecular targets of sensitization of pain pathways in the spinal cord and at how messages arriving in the nervous system from an injured area are modified at the very first synaptic relay. Analyzing the process of synaptic strengthening in the spinal cord in response to

a persistent noxious input has become central to the study of pain sensitization.

There is some logic in the idea that changes at the first synaptic relay in the spinal cord may be critical for the generation of pain hypersensitivity. We know that the spinal cord is not just a simple relay of information such that what comes in must go out, but rather a sophisticated point of integration and modulation such that the message going toward the brain, or the output going toward the muscles, is not a direct reflection of the incoming message. More than 100 years ago, the Scottish surgeon James MacKenzie proposed that impulses arriving in the spinal cord from a diseased organ or from a point of injury would cause a "focus of irritation" in the cord that, owing to its enhanced excitability, would be responsible for increased motor activity, augmented reflexes to other organs, and hypersensitivity to pain caused by transmission of the amplified activity of the "irritable focus" in the spinal cord to the brain. This idea of an "irritable focus" in the spinal cord triggered by messages arriving from a point of disease and generating increased neural excitability leading to pain amplification is an obvious forerunner of the modern concept of central sensitization to pain.

Looking at the relationship between the input that the spinal cord receives from nociceptors in peripheral organs and tissues and the output that spinal-cord neurons send to the brain helps us identify the mechanisms in the cord that amplify pain messages. An interesting biological feature of peripheral nociceptors is that the nerve fibers that transmit their information to the spinal cord are among the thinnest in the nervous system. This imposes severe restrictions on the number of nerve impulses these fibers can transmit and on the maximum frequency of transmission. When we apply intense mechanical stimulation to a nociceptor for two minutes, we notice that the rate at which it sends its message to the brain decreases progressively. This is a physical limitation of the nociceptor's excitability, and there is little we can do about it. However, when we ask people to describe the pain that this stimulus produces we invariably get the answer that there is a progressively increasing pain sensation. If the pain increases as the message from the peripheral nociceptor decreases, the only possible explanation is that there must be mechanisms of amplification in the central nervous system. Several such mechanisms have been detected in the spinal cord. One of them is a phenomenon known as *wind-up*. The name was borrowed from the jargon of baseball, in which is used to describe the motion of the pitcher just before he throws the ball. It evokes a movement of increasing intensity and magnitude.

Wind-up was first detected in the 1960s by scientists who were recording the activity of neurons in the spinal cord and their responses to repetitive stimulation of the sensory nerves at intensities that activated the finest fibers, known to be those concerned with pain transmission. Wind-up is a progressive increase in the magnitude of each response of a spinal-cord neuron to repeated constant-intensity stimuli. The neuron behaves as if it is "winding up" its responses even if the stimulus is kept at a constant level. This is a typical example of the amplification of a message concerned with the transmission of pain-related information. It clearly demonstrated that such amplification can occur at the very first synaptic relay in the spinal cord.

Because wind-up of spinal-cord neurons is relatively easy to detect and even easier to quantify, its discovery produced an explosion of studies that equated it with pain amplification extending the definition of that phenomenon to any detectable kind of amplification, including the activity of a single neuron, the measuring of a withdrawal reflex, and the reported pain sensation of a patient. Although several studies have shown that wind-up isn't always associated with pain perception and that it can also mediate other progressive amplification processes, measuring wind-up remains a popular way to quantify the sensitization process, particularly in the spinal cord.

Looking at the molecular mediators of wind-up and of other similar expressions of hyperexcitability soon revealed that the main culprit was glutamate, one of the most widespread neurotransmitters in the brain and the spinal cord. The hunt for the molecular mechanisms of enhanced excitability in the spinal cord in response to a persistent pain input was then focused on the neural transmission mediated by glutamate and on the various forms and actions of the molecular receptors activated by that neurotransmitter. And here is where the paths of two different functions of the brain, pain and memory, crossed.

Memory is a very enigmatic brain function. As we get older, we appreciate the peculiarities of this most remarkable capacity of the brain more and more. We may be able to remember in great detail events, people, or situations that happened to us 40, 50, or 60 years ago, yet we may find it increasingly difficult to remember where we left our car keys a few hours ago or the name of someone we just met. Memory is a product of synaptic plasticity, which somehow manages to leave permanent traces in our brains associated with events that happened many years ago while failing to store some simple aspects of everyday life. And it seems that a crucial aspect of the formation of memories is the prolonged increase in

excitability that a persistent input to a neuron causes by repeated stimulation, a phenomenon now known as *long-term potentiation* (LTP).

LTP is also a product of glutamate transmission, and the more we know about the mechanisms of pain sensitization the more we believe that they are very similar to those related to the LTP generated in areas of the brain concerned with memory formation. This has led scientists to consider pain sensitization as a kind of *pain memory*, a process whereby a pain perception leaves traces in the brain that contribute to enhanced pain sensitivity when another painful message arrives. The fact that memory and pain hypersensitivity share common molecular mechanisms suggests that the brain deals with these two processes in similar ways. The aim seems to be to retain certain information that can be used to determine a future response, be that a memory or a pain perception.

The strengthening of glutamate-mediated synaptic connections along the pain pathway that generates pain hypersensitivity is a consequence of several elementary mechanisms. These include increases in glutamate release, the work of molecules that maintain the excitability of the neurons once activated by glutamate, and also the mobilization of the receptors for glutamate ("glutamate trafficking"), which makes the transmission of impulses though these synapses easier, more robust, and more persistent. All these processes have been detected in the spinal cord in response to a persistent input from nociceptors and in areas of the brain concerned with the formation of memories.

Glutamate is not the only molecule involved in pain amplification. It has been proposed that many other molecules, transmitters, and modulators play direct or indirect roles in the generation of pain hypersensitivity. One of the most notorious was "Substance P," a molecule that became such a strong candidate for a role in pain perception that many people thought the name stood for *Substance Pain* rather than *Substance Powder* (the more prosaic name given to it in the 1930s by its discoverer, Ulf von Euler). Although much evidence was gathered a few years ago for a role of Substance P in the generation of pain hypersensitivity, clinical trials failed to demonstrate analgesic actions of synthetic drugs that were developed to block its action. But the list of potential players in the process of pain sensitization and hypersensitivity keeps getting longer without any of the candidates taking the definitive role. On the contrary, the more detailed the analysis in molecular terms the more we reach points where many functions coincide, which makes it very difficult to identify a pain-modulating target that wouldn't also interfere with other and equally important functions.

In addition to sensitization (peripheral or central), there is another important mechanism in the amplification of pain sensations: the ability of tactile signals to gain access to pain pathways and cause touch-evoked pain. This happens normally after an injury or inflammation and generates areas of hyperalgesia adjacent to or sometimes remote from the injury site, providing an expanded area of pain hypersensitivity that contributes to guarding the injured body part. But it can also be a feature—sometimes the only feature—of pathological pain in the absence of an originating injury. In all cases it shows that it is possible for tactile and other low-intensity signals to gain access to a pain-generating mechanism in the brain.

One potential mechanism for such an amplification phenomenon is the anatomical or functional reorganization of connections between neurons in the spinal cord and the brain. Most neurons receive inputs from many sources but under some circumstances they may favor only one type—let's say pain. However, in a chronic-pain state or after prolonged painful stimulation these neurons reveal their connectivity to other sensory inputs and can therefore be activated by tactile stimuli as well as by painful stimuli. It is somewhat paradoxical that this analysis, often presented as an alternative to a specificity interpretation of pain pathways, requires as the ultimate step that the activity of a certain neuron be always interpreted by the brain as pain. For this interpretation to work, it is necessary that there be neurons that are always concerned with pain perception. Normally they would be activated only by pain inputs. After an injury, however, they reveal their tactile drives but will still be concerned with pain transmission—an interesting mixture of plasticity at the beginning of the pathway and strict specificity at the other end. The experimental evidence does indeed show that most neurons can express different inputs depending on their degree of excitability, but it also indicates that other neurons have a more robust set of inputs. Anatomical reorganization—meaning the generation of new connections between neurons whereby nerves carrying tactile information grow to contact neurons of the pain pathway—has also been proposed as a mechanism, although the evidence is controversial. This kind of anatomical alteration may occur after major nerve or brain damage but has not been proved to be a mechanism for quick changes in pain sensitivity.

And there are other alternative explanations. Two remarkable features of the generation of pain hypersensitivity are the speed with which it can set in and its dependence on tissue injury (at least under normal circumstances). We all know that it is wise to place a burned finger under a

stream of cold water immediately. This soothes the pain and reduces the area from which we get the burning sensation. The reason is obviously not that we are putting out the fire that burned us; it is that the cold water reduces the excitability of the nerves in the burned area. Exposure to cold is a very good way to decrease the excitability of any cell. Running cold water over a burned finger, or (even better) placing an ice cube on the burned area, reduces the magnitude of the pain message from the point of injury. That, in turn, decreases the hyperexcitability of pain neurons in the spinal cord and the brain and reduces the amount of pain felt as a result of the burn. Next time you burn a finger, try placing an ice cube on the burned area, wait for pain relief, then remove the ice cube. You will notice how quickly the pain comes back. You also will notice touch-evoked pain from a larger area around the finger, the latter being the result of a pain amplification mechanism triggered by your brain. The effect is so rapid that it cannot be due to anatomical reorganization in your brain; it must be due to the modulation of an existing mechanism by the signals arriving from the burned area. And that modulation is expressed by the inhibition your brain applies to the information sent by the finger.

The brain can become hypersensitive to pain either by increasing excitation or by reducing inhibition (the latter is called *disinhibition.*) The inhibition that the brain normally applies to pain perception can be removed by changing the way in which some neurotransmitters work, a mechanism that can explain how a sensation changes from touch to pain. Normally one of the most powerful inhibitory neurotransmitters is gamma-aminobutyric acid (GABA). During persistent painful stimulation, or as a consequence of a nerve lesion, the basic mechanism that makes GABA an inhibitory neurotransmitter changes so that now it becomes an excitatory one. Under normal circumstances, tactile stimuli reduce the transmission of pain signals through the spinal cord by an inhibitory mechanism that uses GABA as the main neurotransmitter. The alteration caused in chronic pain states whereby GABA switches from being inhibitory to being excitatory means that the same tactile stimuli would now activate the pain system rather than inhibit its activity. This mechanism is thought to be the cause for the symptom of touch-evoked pain that is characteristic of many chronic pain states.

A Caveat and a Warning

I will end this chapter with a caveat and a warning. The caveat is that much of what we know about the mechanisms of sensitization and

hypersensitivity in the central nervous system comes from studies restricted to the spinal cord. For about 40 years, the first synaptic relay in the spinal cord has been the main target of studies of pain mechanisms. The warning is that pain is pain only when the brain is involved—that is, pain is in the brain and nowhere else. Of course what happens to the pain message on its way to the brain is important in shaping the information and preparing it for its final processing, but there is still a long way to go from the first synaptic relay to the elaboration of a complex pain perception. Perhaps the obsession with the spinal cord is the reason why, after many years of study, we haven't yet found a therapeutic target for analgesia entirely restricted to a spinal-cord mechanism. The perception of a painful sensation is a brain function, and if we want to understand pain we will have to examine brain mechanisms.

I Feel Your Pain: Perception and the Brain

Between 1930 and 1960, thousands of people were subjected to a surgical procedure that changed their personalities completely. That procedure—called *frontal lobotomy* or, more precisely, *prefrontal leucotomy*—consisted in surgical section of the connections between the frontal lobes of the brain and the rest of the nervous system. The frontal lobes are the most evolved regions of the brain, the bits that distinguish humans from other primates. Severing the connections between the frontal lobes and the rest of the nervous system transformed the patients into undemanding people without drives, passions, or imagination.

Frontal lobotomies were among the surgical interventions aimed at changing peoples' personalities by surgical manipulation of the brain. When first introduced, these procedures (which came to be known as *psychosurgery*) were regarded as highly sophisticated and were welcomed by the medical profession and by the public as a clean and easy way to manage psychotics, people with criminal tendencies, and other unruly creatures. Indeed, frontal lobotomy was developed with the aim of controlling. Its originator, the Portuguese neurologist Antonio Egas Moniz, received the Nobel Prize in 1949 "for his discovery of the therapeutic value of leucotomy in certain psychoses" (to quote the Nobel citation). In the United States, the neurologist Walter Freeman adopted the procedure enthusiastically. Freeman performed more than 2,000 lobotomies, initially on psychotics and later on patients with all sorts of personality disorders and other psychiatric conditions. He developed a quick and easy method of performing a lobotomy—often at the home of the patient, and without general anesthesia—using a simple instrument of his own design. One of Freeman's best-known patients was Rosemary Kennedy, a sister of President John F. Kennedy, who was lobotomized at the age of 23 to treat her mood swings and was left permanently incapacitated.

The main reason for the success and the wide acceptance of such a radical procedure was that at the time there were no other ways to control psychotic behavior. Patients with severe mental disorders were confined to prison-like mental institutions where they spent their entire lives physically restrained. A surgical procedure that transformed these difficult patients into easygoing individuals was a godsend for those who had to deal with them. The ability to change troublesome personalities for the better led to people being lobotomized for all sorts of reasons, some of them not necessarily connected with psychotic or dangerous behavior. The introduction of powerful antipsychotic drugs in the late 1950s reduced and then eliminated the need for this aggressive form of psychosurgery. Indeed, today we regard the wide use of this kind of surgery as unimaginable. But by the end of the 1950s thousands of people were lobotomized, mostly in the United States, in Britain, and in Scandinavia. Studying them yielded deep insights into the workings of the brain.

The main consequence of a frontal lobotomy is a profound change in what we identify as the cognitive functions of the brain: the ability to understand one's place in the universe—both in space and in time—by evaluating the past, assessing the present, and planning for the future. These functions are the hallmark of our species, the very essence of what generates creative thinking, rational decisions, and forward planning. Patients whose frontal lobes are separated from the rest of their brain become dull. Lacking in emotion, they lose will power and are easily distracted. They also lose the ability to make logical plans and rational judgments, can't deal with imaginary situations, and are unable to think things through. They are easily satisfied with immediate gratification, and they don't give much thought to the consequences of their actions. Because they care little about themselves and others, they are easily manipulated and don't cause trouble if challenged. They can be euphoric, agitated, and restless at times, but in most cases they eventually become dull and lifeless. A frontal lobotomy is a straightforward way of eliminating unruly behavior and of controlling difficult personality traits, especially in patients with severe psychosis.

Lobotomy had many unexpected consequences, and one of them had to do with the ability to perceive pain. Psychosurgery was essentially a medical experiment, and physicians were able to study all aspects of brain function on the people that underwent it. Along the way, there were some remarkable discoveries about pain perception.

No Brain, No Pain

In the early days of lobotomy, only psychotic patients were subjected to it. But as more and more people were lobotomized, physicians noticed several profound changes in their neurological profiles. Patients who had been lobotomized didn't complain of pain, even if they had done so before the operation. Careful examination of these patients showed that they hadn't lost the ability to feel pain; their sensory system was intact, and they could detect painful stimuli with the right threshold, quality, and intensity as well as normal people could. However, feeling pain no longer bother them. As with other aspects of their lives, they didn't care much about feeling pain. It didn't worry them or make them unhappy. Lobotomy hadn't abolished the sensation of pain, but it had removed the normal link between pain and suffering. Pain had become a sensory event of little consequence for these people because it didn't make them suffer.

Some physicians thought that lobotomies could be an effective way of dealing with intense pain, especially in patients with terminal cancer and a short life expectancy. Reading the clinical histories of some of the patients who underwent the procedure yields extraordinary insights not only into the suffering of the patient but also into the prevailing culture of the time. Consider two cases described by the American neurologist James Murphy in 1951:

Case 4 A 42-year-old female was reduced to complete incapacitation and dependency upon decreasingly effective hypodermics of opiates, given every hour, because of agonizing pain in the legs. Malignancy of the breast had spread to the lumbosacral spine. Bilateral lobotomy was performed. The patient went through a stormy time because of withdrawal of narcotics and debility, and then recovered sufficiently to become so vituperative and obscene a virago as to result in discharge from hospital at the request of the nursing staff. Two months later, she had become a tractable but outspoken member of society, complaining only of acute pain when her knees were manipulated without warning. She expired four months after surgery.

Case 7 Invasive carcinoma of the pancreas reduced the existence of a 42-year-old white male to hapless dependence upon a morphine-hyoscine mixture which was "like so much water" after three months of two- and three-hourly injection. Bilateral lobotomy was performed through atrophic frontal lobes, with trepidation because of jaundice and low prothrombin levels. Postoperatively, this pillar of society became such a pugnacious practical joker and general social menace as to necessitate firm and abusive talkings-to and the securing of male nursing attendants. Complaints of pain were utilized to plead for mercy re the latest escapade. Eventually (one month), the patient regained equilibrium, and psychic

abnormality persisted only insofar as to make him the "life of the party." Occasional injections of Demerol were sufficient to control discomfort.

In each of these two cases, a lobotomy was performed with the aim of reducing pain. The patients were otherwise psychologically normal, though presumably tormented by intense pain. The elimination of the suffering associated with their pain was offset by a change in behavior that included lack of control. It is very interesting to read what James Murphy thought should be the correct way of dealing with this contrast: "The most effective attitude in caring for the post-lobotomy pain patient is compounded of equal parts of humorous understanding, firmness with what exceeds the bounds of allowable license, and appreciation of the problems of concern to an individual facing early and inevitable death."

Frontal lobotomies for the control of pain are a thing of the past, but they left a legacy. Studies of patients who underwent them demonstrated clearly that the sensory quality of pain and its cognitive consequences are two different processes. The more evolved the brain, the more these cognitive elements influence the overall pain experience. Removing the part of the brain that makes us suffer is sufficient to eliminate pain—at least, to eliminate the kind of pain that makes life miserable. What frontal lobotomies demonstrated—if demonstration ever was necessary—was that the overall experience of pain is one of the highest functions of the brain.

Cognitive Pain

The pain experience has three components. We think of them as inseparable because they always appear together. However, we know that we can tease them out by brain manipulations such as surgery or by the administration of certain drugs. We call these three components *sensory*, *emotional*, and *cognitive*. Let us consider how each of them contributes to the overall pain experience and which regions of the brain deal with each component.

The sensory component is responsible for recognition of the pain sensation. It is the aspect of pain most directly linked to what we call *nociception*: the detection of harmful or potentially harmful stimuli. It is also, in evolutionary terms, the oldest function associated with pain: the ability to sense danger and trigger a defensive reaction to it. It is probably all that many animals, especially invertebrates and simpler vertebrates, have as a pain experience.

The sensory component of pain is the *ouch!* component. It tells us that harm has occurred or that harm will occur if the stimulus persists and compels us (usually by a reflex action) to avoid or flee from the source of the injury. Its origin is in the peripheral sensors for the detection of injury that all animals, including humans, have in the skin, the muscles, the joints, and the internal organs. Messages from these nociceptors reach the spinal cord and the brain through a relatively simple chain of neurons and reach the sensory cortex of the brain, where they are resolved into a sensory experience of pain. In this respect, the sensory component of pain is similar to those of vision or hearing.

The second component of the pain experience is the emotional or affective reaction to it. In normal humans this is always an aversive and unpleasant emotional response. Our sensory brain tells us that an injury has occurred, and our emotional brain makes us unhappy and triggers aversive reactions. The emotional component of the pain experience also tells us that there is more to pain than the simple detection of injury: pain makes us cry, changes our heart rate and respiration, affects the regulation of our internal organs, and gives us a deep feeling of unpleasantness and a strong aversion to the whole process. The emotional component is the *get rid of my pain!* component.

The emotional reactions to pain are distributed among many parts of the brain, including the brain stem, the hypothalamus, regions concerned with hormonal regulation, the amygdala, and the anterior cingulate cortex. The common feature of all the emotions triggered by pain is the feeling of unpleasantness and the aversive nature of the emotional reaction. There are, however, differences between emotions associated with anxiety—more characteristic of acute pain states—and those that generate depressive feelings—a consequence of chronic pain. We believe that other primates and other higher vertebrates also have emotional reactions to pain, as their reactions to complex pain experiences aren't so different from ours. But to what extent the emotions of a cat, a dog, or a chimpanzee are similar to the emotions we feel is a matter of debate.

The third component of pain, and the one most typically human, is the cognitive component. Not only do we feel the pain and show an instinctive aversive reaction to it; we also worry about its meaning. We want to know why we feel pain, what it means to our survival and our future, and how it may affect our lives and the lives of people close to us. We want to know whether it will go away soon and how it will influence our work, our social life. Is it serious? Am I going to die? Will I be able to walk

again, or to play with my children? What is going on? The cognitive component of pain is the *why?* component.

This kind of cognitive function is the product of the frontal lobes of our brains, which in order to function properly must have good connections with the emotional and sensory areas of the brain. The cognitive component of pain requires self-consciousness (a capacity to understand our place in the universe, knowledge that our lives have a beginning and an end and that our death will influence other people's lives). We can be fairly sure that pain cognition is a uniquely human experience.

To understand how the three components of the pain experience interact, consider a couple of examples. First, think of yourself happily playing with your children on a beach on a glorious sunny day. Suddenly you step on a hidden piece of glass from a broken bottle and cut your foot badly. There is bleeding, and there is a lot of sensory pain. In addition, you feel bad because your happy moment has been interrupted, you curse the person who left the bottle behind, and you feel anxious about the whole experience. Your emotional pain kicks in. But then you look at the wound and see that it isn't really bad. The bleeding soon stops, and you may not need stitches. Thus, it is really nothing, it will not affect the rest of your vacation, it may be a good excuse to stop playing with your kids and have a break, and you may get some sympathy from your family. Cognition has taken over and now colors the entire pain experience. The sensory pain is still there, and it is pretty intense, but there really isn't anything to worry about.

Now consider a second example. For a few weeks you have felt a dull pain in your abdomen. Though not very strong, it bothers you enough that you go to a physician, who, ominously, suggests a lot of tests. You go from clinic to clinic and from specialist to specialist, each of whom looks gloomier than the last. Your sensory pain isn't intense, but your emotions are running riot and you can't sleep well at night. Eventually the dreaded verdict is delivered: you have an intestinal cancer, a particularly nasty form. The physicians are all very sorry and supportive, but they tell you that there is little they can do and that you don't have much longer to live. The sensory pain is not so strong; in fact it may be less intense than what you felt when you cut your foot. But emotions are now controlling your life. The cognitive realization that you are going to die soon, leaving your family behind, makes the overall pain experience much more unpleasant and unbearable than the more intense but less worrisome event at the beach.

Cognitive pain is what transforms pain into suffering. It is a function of the most evolved regions of our brains—the regions directly associated with memory, self-consciousness, rational thought, and other high brain functions. Ultimately, it is cognition that will determine the overall intensity of a pain experience. We need to rationalize and understand the cause and course of our pain. When unable to do so, we need others—the medical profession—to do it for us. The relationship between a patient and a physician hinges on the patient's cognitive need to understand what is wrong and the physician's ability to provide a suitable explanation and treatment.

A frontal lobotomy removes the cognitive component from the overall pain experience. Lobotomized patients still feel sensory pain, and can have some emotional unpleasant reactions to it, but the pain no longer bothers them. And that is as good as analgesia, for a pain that doesn't bother you loses its capacity to make you suffer. It is very hard for most of us to think of the three components of the pain experience separately, since they appear together and are intimately linked to one another in all situations. How does a sensory pain feel when it doesn't bother you? Can you have an emotional unpleasant reaction to pain yet not worry about what it means for your survival? A frontal lobotomy might help you understand these distinctions, but don't try that at home. Some drugs, most notably the opiates, also dissociate the sensory from the cognitive pain.

Thus, in the end, all pain is in the brain. The overall pain experience requires cognition and is a consequence of rational thought, one of the most evolved functions of our brains and the one that makes us characteristically human. It is remarkable that pain, a sensory process that began in simple animals as a reflex function to avoid trouble, has evolved into suffering, one of the highest and most complex functions of the human brain.

Seeing Pain

As was discussed in previous chapters, the prevailing model of brain function is that of a network of neurons connected through pathways made up by the projections of the neurons. This model has generated a switchboard-like notion of brain function: signals start in a sense organ and, through a series of pathways and connections, messages flow through the network in charge of a specific function, be that pain, vision, or posture control. As far as pain is concerned, this model is the natural

consequence of an idea originally proposed by Descartes in the seventeenth century: pull a string from a site of injury and a bell rings in the brain. But although the model can work well for the detection of injury and for the initial processing of pain signals in the spinal cord, it fails to help us understand pain perception at the brain level.

The experience of pain is multi-dimensional, sensory, emotional, and cognitive, and it is very likely that many regions of the brain are simultaneously active when pain is felt. And not only is this true for the normal acute pain felt after an injury; it is also true (and even more so) for the chronic pain of a long-lasting disease or for abnormal pain sensations generated by a dysfunctional brain. The classical connectivity model needs to be modified to take into account simultaneous activations of various brain regions whose contributions to the overall activity generate the individual pain experience. This is a distributed model of parallel processing—with several things being done at the same time—leading to associations between different patterns of activation of brain regions for a particular pain experience. It is a model that Ron Melzack, a prominent figure in the modern study of pain mechanisms, has described as a "pain matrix" or a "neuromatrix." Each pain experience will have a neurosignature of brain activation that will carry the sensory, emotional, and cognitive elements of the pain state.

Can we detect neurosignatures and associate them with particular pain experiences? The process would be like recording a patient's electrocardiogram and then diagnosing a cardiac disease on the basis of a consistent pattern of abnormal waves in the recording. A similar procedure for pain would offer an objective tool with which to measure pain and to identify the intensity of a pain-producing condition. Pain would no longer be a subjective feeling; it would be a variable that could be measured objectively—a boon for patients, for pain physicians, and especially for medical insurance companies and health-care systems.

In the last few years, a strong current of opinion has developed that this dream may be realized by means of brain imaging. For a very long time, physicians and scientists have tried to obtain images of the brain from patients or from human volunteers and then to correlate the specific alterations observed in these images with changes in brain function or with neurological diseases. Older techniques were based on the use of x-rays of the head adding radio opaque contrast into the cavities of the brain or through the blood vessels but the results were very limited and generally unsatisfactory. In the last two or three decades there have been substantial advances in the technology of brain imaging thanks to

the use of computers that can quickly process thousands of images and the use of techniques such as magnetic resonance, detection of changes in blood flow through brain regions, and the measurement of weak radioactive substances that bind to specific brain regions. These techniques, which are always improving, have added fascinating observations to our knowledge of brain function. We can now literally see how the brain is activated, not only by external stimuli, but also by changes in emotional states, by mental activity, or even by the recalling of events. We are getting closer to the age-old fantasy of being able to read people's minds.

There are essentially two kinds of modern brain imaging: anatomical and functional. Anatomical brain imaging yields very detailed images of the brain and provides information about the sizes of various brain features and about the presence of anatomical abnormalities, such as tumors, dead tissue, blood clots, or hemorrhages. It is an extremely useful tool for assessing the structural elements of the brain. Functional brain imaging, on the other hand, yields information about how the brain works when undertaking physical or mental tasks, which regions are activated by external stimuli, and what patterns of activity correspond to various sensory and motor states. A combination of functional and anatomical techniques gives a complete picture of the brain activity generated in response to an external stimulus or of the brain activity generated by introspection and internal mental processes.

Brain-imaging studies of pain states in both normal human volunteers and pain patients have generated two important pieces of knowledge. The first is that many regions of the brain are active simultaneously during a pain experience. The second is that chronic pain is associated with structural changes of the brain, and that pain can literally change your brain.

Let us first consider the information that has emerged from brain imaging of normal volunteers who were subjected to painful stimuli or painful events. As would be expected, a brief painful stimulus, such as heat applied to the hand or a pinch of a finger, activates the somatosensory cortex, a region of the outermost portion of gray matter that covers the brain and that receives and integrates all sensory events from the body. This is the closest we get to the ringing bell in Descartes' model: the final destination of a relatively simple and straightforward pathway that detects injury and transmits the signals directly to the brain. But two other important areas of the brain—the anterior insular cortex and the anterior cingulate cortex—are also turned on by these acute

painful stimuli, and their activities correlate best with the emotional and cognitive components of the pain experience. These two areas belong to the prefrontal cortex—a region of the brain adjacent to the frontal lobes, the most evolved part of the human brain.

The anterior insular cortex was once thought to be concerned with the processing of sensations from internal organs—not only sensations of gastric or intestinal distension, but also those of other complex internal feelings, such as orgasm or tiredness. Imaging studies have shown this region to be active during sensory events associated with emotional and affective feelings, such as motherly love or craving certain foods. Likewise, the anterior cingulate cortex is active as a result of emotional events, but in this case it seems that the association is negative, dealing with the unpleasantness and aversive components of the pain experience. Both areas are essential for mental processes that include error awareness, decision making, and self-recognition. It would seem that these brain areas integrate the emotional component of a pain experience and provide a link between the emotional and the cognitive elements of pain perception.

Brain areas normally associated with reward and sensory control can also be activated by painful stimuli. We think these areas are involved in the modulation of a painful experience, a process that can be triggered by external events or stress or can be internally generated as a placebo response. These questions of pain modulation will be discussed in another chapter, but is important to point out here that a relatively simple acute painful stimulus applied to a normal human volunteer triggers activity in virtually the entire brain.

Earlier in the book it was mentioned that extreme views of brain localization of individual functions led to the pseudo-science of phrenology. Critics of the data generated by brain imaging have warned that it may lead to a modern phrenology, with various regions of the brain labeled as the seats of complex mental activities. The combination of sophisticated imaging technology and very smart experimental protocols tends to encourage interpretations of the brain based on the identification of individual functions to restricted brain areas, a kind of high-tech phrenology. Yet the most important observations to have come from brain-imaging studies is that many brain regions are simultaneously active during a pain experience and that most of them are also active during other tasks that share emotional and cognitive components with the perception of pain. Humans have a tendency to use a linear thought process when approaching every question, and it is hard to think in terms

of being able to do many things at the same time to produce an overall result. But this is the way the brain seems to work: by generating mental states that are the consequences of variable patterns of coexisting activity in several brain regions at any moment. It is the opposite of a strict localization approach.

Brain imaging has also been used to study chronic-pain patients. On the functional side, the results that have emerged from these studies show changes in the intensity of the activation of brain regions normally turned on by pain, differential involvement of these regions in the overall pain response, and abnormal activation of some brain areas. Each abnormality detected with brain-imaging is related to the specific chronic-pain disease, which reinforces the view that one day we may be able to use brain imaging to diagnose pain in the same way that we now use an electrocardiogram to diagnose heart disease. But the most spectacular results to emerge from recent brain-imaging studies of chronic pain are that the brains of the patients are structurally abnormal and that chronic pain is associated with anatomically detectable changes in them. This was first detected in patients suffering from chronic low-back pain. Images of the brains of these patients showed a reduction in the gray matter of the thalamus (an important sensory region) but also showed a reduction in the gray matter of the prefrontal cortex (the area associated with the emotional and cognitive aspects of the pain experience). Further studies have shown similar structural changes in patients suffering from various forms of chronic pain, including neuropathic pain, irritable bowel syndrome, fibromyalgia, and even headaches. Most of the changes are in the form of reduced amounts of gray matter in the areas of the brain normally activated by pain, particularly those that integrate emotional and cognitive elements. In a few cases, increased gray matter in some of these regions has also been detected in chronic-pain patients. The common feature is a structural alteration, usually in the form of a reduction of gray matter, in areas of the brain that deal with the pain experience. But there is also some variation among the various chronic-pain diseases: the specific pattern of alterations varies from pain condition to pain condition.

In addition, biochemical alterations have been found in chronic-pain patients, including reduced levels of serotonin and dopamine—two neurotransmitters that participate in the elaboration of reward responses. Together with the structural alterations, these observations are evidence of profound changes in the brains of patients suffering from chronic-pain diseases. This leads to two obvious questions: Are these alterations causes

of the chronic-pain state, or are the consequences of it? Since the brains of chronic-pain patients are abnormal, can we detect other neurological or psychiatric problems associated with chronic-pain diseases?

The answer to the first question is not known. It may be that the chronic-pain condition causes structural changes in the brain. It is also possible that a primary brain alteration may cause the chronic-pain state. However, successful treatment of the pain has been shown to reduce or reverse the structural changes; this would argue in favor of pain's being the primary cause of the brain alterations. What is certain is that a chronic-pain state goes hand in hand with detectable structural and bio-chemical changes in the brain, which further supports the view that imaging may soon be an objective tool for detecting or even measuring the magnitude of chronic pain.

The answer to the second question is Yes. Chronic pain is associated with psychiatric conditions (e.g. depression and chronic anxiety), and patients suffering from chronic pain show cognitive impairments consistent with altered brain function, including decreases in working memory and deficits in decision making. The latter have been detected in a series of studies of chronic-pain patients in which their capacity to make the right decision was assessed by means of a gambling test. It was found that subjects suffering from chronic pain tended to prefer immediate and larger rewards that in the long term would lead to an overall loss over rewards that were smaller in the short term but would lead to long-term gains. It is significant that chronic-pain patients preferred short-term rewards over long-term gains. It seems that chronic pain enhances the need for an immediate reward—pain relief—at any cost and militates against the more logical choice of a long-term gain.

Pain Neurons

Brain imaging makes it possible to see how the whole brain reacts to a painful event and how chronic pain alters its structure and its functioning. But the brain is made up of billions of nerve cells whose activity is directly related to what the brain ultimately does, and we don't know whether there are individual neurons in the brain that are concerned only with processing pain-related events or how the activity of such neurons would ultimately lead to a pain experience.

Much of what we know about pain neurons in the brain comes from reports by neurosurgeons, who take advantage of their access to the human brain to explore it during operations. One of the pioneering surgeons was Wilder Penfield, who in the mid 1930s founded the Montreal

Neurological Institute at McGill University. Penfield was not only an accomplished neurosurgeon but also a neuroscientist with a keen interest in the workings of the brain, which he pursued by training with some of the giants of neuroscience of his time, including Sherrington and Ramón y Cajal. He developed a procedure for treating epilepsy that was based on making restricted lesions in the areas of the brain where the epileptic attacks began. The patients remained conscious during the procedure, under local anesthesia, so Penfield could stimulate various points on the surface of the brain with low-intensity electrical currents and ask the patients what they felt, or could observe their movements and behavior.

Penfield's pioneering work produced maps of the areas of the brain that integrate sensory experiences and motor reactions. Except for a few sketchy observations, all the sensations reported by Penfield's patients were non-painful. But his experimental approach is still in use today, and many other neurosurgeons have added further observations using similar and more refined techniques. The use of brain imaging to identify the areas of the brain that are activated by painful stimuli has also contributed to better targeting during surgery. We now know that stimulation of focal points of the prefrontal cortex, including the anterior cingulate cortex and regions of the insula, evokes feelings of pain in conscious patients.

There are two kinds of painful experience that can be evoked by brain stimulation. The first type is a pure sensory experience of pain. It is most commonly generated by stimulating points along the sensory pathway that carries injury-related information, including some areas of the thalamus (the main sensory nucleus of the brain) and of the somatosensory cortex. The second type of experience is a pain feeling whose principal characteristic is unpleasantness that generates an aversive emotional response in the patient. Experiences of the second kind are typically evoked by stimulation of prefrontal areas, including the insula and the anterior cingulate cortex.

What brain-stimulation studies show is that there must be neurons in the brain whose primary task is to process pain experiences, either purely sensory or with added emotional or cognitive components. The search for such neurons has been carried out experimentally by recording the electrical activity of individual nerve cells in conscious laboratory animals and correlating the neuron's activity with the animal's behavioral reactions. These studies have demonstrated that neurons activated by painful stimuli are present in several areas of the brain, that those in primarily sensory regions—thalamus and somatosensory cortex—give time-locked

responses to painful stimuli, and that those in associative areas of the brain show more complex activity, often modulated by other sensory inputs or by distraction and reward.

The data from animal studies led neurosurgeons to look for pain-related neuronal activity in the areas that had been identified in the laboratory. In addition, information obtained by imaging the human brain during pain states gave clues as to what regions of the brain should be explored during surgical procedures. It is now possible to record the electrical activity of single neurons in a conscious human during brain surgery as well as to produce very localized stimulation of these neurons, and either of these methods allows direct correlations to be made between the activity of individual nerve cells and the verbal reports of the patient during the procedure.

Nerve cells activated by painful stimuli have been found in many regions of the human brain, including primary sensory pathways and associative areas. Their responses can be complex and inconsistent and are often modulated by the emotional state of the patient and by other sensory stimuli. On the other hand, restricted stimulation of small areas of the brain has been shown to evoke feelings of pain ranging from the simplest form of painful sensation to complex experiences, including referred pain, memory of pain sensations that occurred long before, phantom-limb pain, and angina. Often these complex experiences are accompanied by emotional reactions, which can be intense enough to generate extreme anxiety or even panic.

The search for pain neurons in the human brain has confirmed the locations of the areas and regions where pain sensations are integrated and has yielded some insights into the complexity of the overall pain experience. Unfortunately, we are still very far from being able to correlate patterns of activity in individual neurons with complex mental states, and it is hard to see that this would ever be possible with current techniques. I opened this chapter with some comments on how a gross procedure such as a frontal lobotomy was instrumental in demonstrating the essential role of the frontal lobes of our brains in the process that transforms sensory pain into suffering. We know that eliminating suffering also eliminates pain, and we know where in the brain this transformation occurs. But we remain ignorant of the biological mechanisms that link brain activity with consciousness. We are able to manipulate this link, and in doing so we can modify pain perception, but we don't really know the fundamental process that mediates the relationship between brain activity and sensory perception.

7 A Certain Gut Feeling: Visceral Pain

Visceral pain is pain from the inside of the body, a sensation that originates from the internal organs and tissues. It is by far the most common
cause of pain. Everyone has experienced pain from an upset stomach or
an intestinal infection. The pain of passing a kidney stone (a small piece
of precipitated urinary salts) from the kidney to the bladder is excruciating. Many people suffer from a kind of cardiac pain called *angina*, a word
derived from the Latin word *angor*, meaning *anxiety* or *anguish*, a testa-
ment to its extreme unpleasantness. We inflict severe pain on our mothers
during childbirth, a pain that originates from contractions and distensions of the uterus and the cervix. And throughout their reproductive
years many women suffer from menstrual cramps that disturb their lives
every four weeks.

On first examination, it would appear that visceral pain is a physiological kind of pain, a part of our sensory repertoire, a normal function
of the brain that signals that something is wrong inside us and that
we should do something about it. In this respect, visceral pain is not
different from the pain we feel when we sustain an injury to an external
body part. Or is it? Some internal organs, including the uterus and the
bladder, can be sources of considerable pain; others, such as the liver
and the spleen, hurt very little or not at all. Extensive damage to the
lungs is virtually painless, but contractures of the ureter or the intestine,
even if they will not cause injury, are intensely painful. And why should
a normal process such as childbirth be so painful? Very often there is
no relation between internal injury and pain. If visceral pain is a protective component of our sensory repertoire, there should be a logical
explanation for its presence and its intensity. If you burn a finger, the
mechanisms of your brain cause you to draw the finger away from the
fire, and the pain teaches you not to put it near a fire again. It would
be absurd to feel pain when you burn a finger but not when you burn

a toe or a leg. In order to be protective, pain has to be rational and persuasive.

Why do we feel visceral pain? We know that "Why?" isn't a good question to ask in biology; the answer invariably is "We are made that way." But we can ask why we feel visceral pain the way we do, and what such pain means for the survival of the individual and of the species. Is visceral pain protective? If it is, what is this pain protecting us from? Does it have any survival value? Can we tell when a pain from our internal organs is useful and when it is pathological? Should we do something about reducing or even avoiding visceral pain in the same way that we avoid injury to our skin or to our muscles?

Mankind has been asking these questions from the beginning of time, puzzled by the illogical nature of many forms of visceral pain and trying to find meaning to a kind of pain that often defies explanation. For instance, why is childbirth painful? We have a powerful mechanism that encourages us to perpetuate our species via by a pleasurable process but the act of giving birth is painful and unpleasant. This doesn't make much sense. As a medical student in the 1960s, when obstetric analgesia was very limited, I remember witnessing the pain of many women giving birth and hearing their pledges that this would be their last child. This isn't the best way of going about perpetuating our species.

In the Judeo-Christian tradition, the pain of childbirth is God's curse on all women for Eve's original sin: "In sorrow thou shalt bring forth children" (Genesis 3:16). This shows that people have been puzzled about the meaning of visceral pain for a long time. The pain of childbirth is not a pain that you may or may not have; it is part of your normal biology; but it doesn't make any sense, and therefore it was attributed to a supernatural curse. In the late nineteenth century, when obstetric analgesia was first introduced to reduce the pain of childbirth, there was a strong movement against this kind of pain relief on the grounds that it was against God's will. Progress has always encountered such obstacles.

We can try to explain the meaning and usefulness of visceral pain by looking at its clinical signs and properties and by identifying the organs that generate painful sensations and the range of sensations that can be evoked from them. Analysis of the brain mechanisms of visceral pain is a powerful tool with which to gain insight into its significance. Visceral pain shows five clinical characteristics that are very different from those of pain from the skin, the muscles, or the joints:

Some internal organs don't hurt when injured or damaged.

There is no clear relation between injury to an internal organ and pain.

Visceral pain is often felt in areas of the body other than the organ where the pain originates.

Visceral pain is very diffuse and badly localized.

Pain from internal organs is always accompanied by exaggerated reactions, such as tense or contracted muscles, changes in blood pressure, heavy breathing, or sweating.

Let us examine in some detail each one of these special properties.

Not All Internal Organs Hurt

One reason why lung cancer is often fatal is that it is virtually painless until it is too late to do anything about it. Most liver diseases, including cirrhosis and some other substantial degenerative disorders, are essentially painless. Yet distensions of the tubes that connect the gall bladder with the liver, or of the ureters that connect the kidneys to the bladder, are excruciatingly painful even when the damage to the organs is relatively small. Likewise, distensions or contractions of the uterus generate a deep and aching pain, but damage to the ovaries is painless. There doesn't seem to be any logic to the fact that some internal organs hurt and others don't.

Many years ago, it was thought that the reason for this strange state of affairs was that some internal organs were not innervated—that they lacked the nerve sensors necessary to pick up the signs of damage and transmit them to the brain. However, we now know that this is not the case. Every internal organ has sensory innervation that is always picking up signals and transmitting the information to the brain. The sensory innervation of our internal organs is, in principle, not very different from the sensory innervation of the skin, the muscles, or the joints. There is, however, one very important difference. In the case of the skin, the muscles, and the joints, every signal picked up and transmitted to the brain by sensory nerves has the potential to become part of a conscious sensory perception directly related to the properties of the stimulus that generated the signals. If an object comes into contact with your skin, sensory nerves record the force of the contact, the temperature of the object, and the velocity and acceleration of the impact and send this information to your brain, where, in addition to the reactions that will be set in motion to deal with the event, you will perceive a clear sensation of the shape, force, and temperature of the object in question. The situation in the internal organs is quite different. The liver, for instance, contains numerous sensors that detect the osmotic pressure of the blood

that circulates through it, the concentration of glucose in this blood, the intra-hepatic pressure, and many other such events. This information is sent to the brain and used for physiological regulation of the liver's function. The brain generates signals that control the variables responsible for blood circulation through the liver, glucose absorption and concentration, and many other aspects of liver function, all without any conscious perception of these processes. Much of the sensory traffic from internal organs to the brain never reaches consciousness, and therefore no sensations originate from these organs.

Some sensory signals from certain organs do reach consciousness and generate sensory experiences of pain and discomfort. These are the organs that hurt, such as the gut, the bladder, or the uterus. The properties of their sensory nerves and the ability of these nerves to activate mechanisms in the brain that will reach consciousness determine the type of sensations elicited from any particular organ. If an organ doesn't have sensory nerves capable of activating conscious perceptions, it will seem to be painless. If an organ does have such sensory nerves, it will be capable of hurting. Every internal organ has sensory innervation, but only those whose sensors are capable of generating conscious perceptions will be sources of pain and discomfort. A great deal of the traffic toward the brain from our internal organs goes unnoticed because it is mainly concerned with physiological regulations. That is just as well. Mercifully, we aren't constantly being made aware of the osmotic pressure inside our liver, the accuracy of our pancreatic function, or the efficiency of the secretions in our stomach.

Which organs are sensitive and capable of generating conscious sensations, and which organs aren't? More important, are there characteristics that would explain why some organs hurt and others don't, a distinction that doesn't appear to be related to the survival value of the sensation?

One such characteristic is whether or not the organ in question is hollow. Most solid organs (*parenchymatous* organs, in medical jargon) are insensitive to pain or to any kind of sensory perception. These include the liver, the kidneys, the spleen, the lungs, and the ovaries (but not the testicles). Hollow organs from which pain is the only sensation that can be evoked include the ureters, the gall bladder, the gall-bladder ducts, the trachea, and the bronchia. Those with a range of sensations from distension to pain include the entire length of the gut from the esophagus to the rectum, the bladder, the uterus, and the vagina.

The distinction between hollow organs that hurt and solid organs that don't hurt is not trivial. Every hollow organ is connected to the external

environment through a natural orifice, and therefore the lining of the hollow cavity is not a part of our internal environment but an interface between the external and the internal environments. Nowhere is this more apparent than in the gut. What goes through the inside of the gut is what we put in it, whether nutritious food or anything else (healthy or unhealthy) that we care to ingest. It can be hot or cold, and it can contain objects capable of injuring the gut or even poisoning and killing us; the lining of the gut is as much a barrier to the external environment as is the skin. Even under normal circumstances, the contents of our guts have chemical properties that would make them toxic or even lethal if they were to come into contact with our internal environment. Stomach acid, the digestive enzymes of the small intestine, and the bacterial flora of the large intestine are good examples of stuff we don't want to penetrate the lining of our intestines. Likewise, the inside of the bladder and the inside of the ureter are connected with the external environment, and their content (urine) is a product of excretion with a chemical composition that would make it very dangerous if it were to come into contact with our internal environment.

Pain is a protective sensation that defends the organism against a hostile external environment right at the interface where the hostilities occur (the skin, the muscles, the joints), but also at other interfaces with the external environment: such as the linings of the gut, of the bladder, and of the reproductive organs. We have a simple but effective alarm system that warns us when we eat something that will injure us, or when an inflammatory reaction defends us from intruders. Such an alarm system didn't develop in solid organs, which aren't part of our interface with the external environment, and their sensory innervation remains dedicated to controlling their functions without reaching the level of consciousness.

It is often said that the only sensation we can get from our internal organs is that of pain, ranging from mild discomfort to excruciating agony. However, some hollow organs also are sources of non-painful sensations—most commonly fullness or distension that drives us to take immediate action to empty the organ. Conscious control of micturition and defecation begins with an initial feeling of distension and an urge to empty the bladder or the gut. If it is socially appropriate to do so, we can take care of these bodily functions; if it isn't, the feeling of fullness quickly develops into an unpleasant sensation that rapidly progresses to pain. Even sensations of fullness of the bladder or the rectum, not generally considered painful, are only the beginning of a sensory process that

will move toward pain if the distension continues and the organ in question isn't emptied. As we will see later in the chapter, this is due to special properties of the neural sensors that signal distension in the hollow organs.

There are two apparent exceptions to the rule that only hollow organs hurt: the testicles and the heart. As every man knows, the testicles can be a source of extremely painful sensations as a consequence of mechanical impact, torsion, pressure, or inflammation. The nerve sensors that signal testicular pain aren't located inside the testes themselves but in the connective tissue around them. These sensors are known to respond to mechanical and thermal stimuli and increase their responses during inflammation. They are in all respects, pain sensors or nociceptors. During fetal development the testicles (like the ovaries) are internal organs, but just before birth they descend into the scrotum, where they are about six degrees Celsius cooler than they would have been inside the abdomen; the lower temperature helps the production of fertile sperm. They become external features, and their sensory innervation protects them from injury.

The case of the heart is quite different. The heart is a highly specialized muscle that shares many features with the rest of the muscles of the body, including the properties of its sensory innervation. Its pain receptors are exquisitely sensitive to reductions in blood flow and to the chemicals produced by ischemia, particularly under cardiac strain. Pain from the heart is always produced by a reduction in the flow of blood through the cardiac tissue, which leads to activation of cardiac pain receptors. The resulting sensation—commensurate with the seriousness of the originating stimulus—is one of chest oppression and impending death. It is somewhat similar to the sensations of cramping that occur when the flow of blood to other muscles is reduced. Cardiac pain is a powerful alarm signal that forces a person to reduce his or her activity, but it is not a component of a normal pain repertoire. When cardiac pain occurs, it is always a sign of a sick heart and of a compromised blood flow that requires repair, not merely reduction of activity.

The Relationship between Injury and Pain in Internal Organs

We are accustomed to thinking that pain is produced by injury and that injury invariably leads to pain. This holds true for the skin, the muscles, the joints, and the somatic organs, but not for the visceral organs. Many forms of injury to internal organs are painless, whereas forms of stimula-

tion to internal organs that don't cause injury can produce pain. This is attributable to special properties of the sensory nerves that supply internal organs.

How do we know so much about the relationship between injury and pain, especially of our internal organs? There was a time, not long ago, when surgery was performed without anesthesia. If you were lucky you would be offered a swig of an alcoholic beverage. Legs would be sawn off and bellies opened by surgeons whose skills consisted mainly of being able to operate quickly and knowing what hurts and what doesn't. This state of affairs changed with the introduction of safe general and local anesthetics in the last 100 years—something for which to be grateful to pain scientists and clinicians.

Surgeons who opened abdomens knew that cutting the skin and the muscle was very painful, but that once you were inside the belly there were many things that you could do without causing any pain. Some organs, including the liver and the kidneys, were completely insensitive. Even internal organs that were sensitive to pain, such as the intestines and the stomach, could be cut or burned with a cautery without the patient reporting any pain. There was no relation between the injury produced in these organs and the perception of pain. Conversely, surgeons knew that twisting or stretching of the intestine, sustained contracture of the intestinal muscle, or over-distension of the gut invariably generated strong complaints, even though there was no apparent injury. In these cases there was no relation between the perception of pain and the presence of an injury in the internal organ.

What determines the range of sensations that we can feel from any part of our bodies, and the relation of these sensations to the various kinds of stimuli, is the properties of the sensors that innervate our bodies. An alarm in your house wouldn't be able to detect an intruder if it weren't connected to a camera or to a motion detector. Likewise, your alarm system—pain—depends critically on the type of sensors that detect and send to the brain information about what is going on in every part of your body. The properties and characteristics of the sensors in our internal organs determine which stimuli cause pain and which don't. If cutting or burning an internal organ doesn't cause pain or any other sensation, we can safely assume that the organ doesn't have sensors that would encode these forms of stimulation, or that whichever sensors are activated by these stimuli don't send signals to areas of the brain where conscious perceptions are processed and integrated. On the other hand, if non-injury-producing stimuli such as stretching or

distension evoke intense pain, it follows that the organ in question possesses sensors that can encode such stimuli, and that their activation sends information to the brain that is processed as pain. The appropriate relationship must therefore be established between the properties of the sensor and the sensation that their activation generates, and not between injury and pain. This is particularly important when discussing visceral pain.

Visceral pain sensors (called *visceral nociceptors* in the medical literature) share some characteristics with pain sensors in the skin, the muscles, and the joints, but they also have some special properties that determine the clinical features of visceral pain. Most visceral nociceptors are highly sensitive to ischemia (a reduction or lack of blood flow to the tissue) and to the tissue chemicals released by stressed cells as a consequence of reduced blood flow. They are also very sensitive to the products of inflammation, which, in combination with their sensitivity to ischemia, makes them excellent sensors of local alterations in an organ associated with irritation, changes in blood flow, and inflammation, all of which can generate persistent pain sensations in (for example) the gut or the bladder. The ability of visceral nociceptors to increase their sensitivity as a consequence of inflammation, even when the inflammatory process remains subclinical, is believed to be the cause of disorders in which pain from an internal organ is felt in the absence of clinically demonstrable alteration of that organ. Increased sensitivity—sensitization—of visceral nociceptors can account for such functional pain states.

Many visceral sensory receptors, whether or not they signal pain or are involved in the control of the functions of internal organs, are sensitive to mechanical stimuli. This property is especially noticeable in the sensors located in organs with substantial muscle layers (e.g., the gut or the bladder) whose functioning requires a strong motor component (e.g., the propulsion of the contents of the gut or the storage of urine and the emptying of the bladder). These visceral sensors are activated by distension of the organ or by changes in tension in the wall of the organ, and take part in both the control of the motility of the internal organ and the transmission to the brain of sensory signals that lead to conscious perception of fullness and to contractions of the organ. An important feature of these sensors is their ability to have a stimulus-response function (the relationship between the intensity of a stimulus and the response of the sensor) that encodes the full range of mechanical events from non-painful to painful. The sensory innervation of the skin, the muscles, and the joints includes sensors that fall into different categories depending

on whether their encoding ranges span only innocuous or only noxious intensities of stimulation. Yet in the viscera, and especially in hollow organs with important motor components, most mechanically sensitive sensors progressively increase their responses as the stimulus moves from an innocuous distension to a noxious one.

Sensors that encode low-intensity and high-intensity stimuli are also present in internal organs, and they probably are concerned with the sensing of normal physiological events and of noxious events, respectively. The intensity-encoding sensors constitute a special category of sensors. They probably are concerned with the signaling of events that begin as innocuous and move to noxious — that is, with the sort of stimuli that, if applied to the bladder or the rectum, would generate an initial sensation of fullness that would progress to discomfort if the organ weren't emptied. Such sensors have also been detected in the esophagus (from which we can get initial sensations of fullness leading to pain), but not in the ureter or the gall bladder (from which we can only get sensations of pain). In these cases, the pain signal is entirely mediated by high-threshold nociceptors that are activated only by large increases in distension pressure, which are always painful.

Referred Visceral Pain

At the peak of high drama in a typical Hollywood movie, a middle-aged man suffers a heart attack. In addition to his convincing and well-rehearsed expression of pain, the actor grabs his left arm in a gesture of considerable pain. His face illustrates the magnitude of his pain with an expression that shows the intensity of his anguish. Since he also grabs his left arm, we all know, without a doubt, that it is a heart attack. If the character had been shot in his right shoulder, the actor would have grabbed that shoulder; if the character had broken a leg, the pain would have been in that leg, if an ankle had been twisted, it would have been in that ankle. How is it that when the heart is the source of the pain it is felt in the left arm?

The phenomenon in which a sensation is felt in a part of the body other than the one in which the pain originates is called *referred pain*. Referred pain is not exclusive to pain from internal organs. Some forms of muscle pain are also referred. However, referred pain is so characteristic of visceral pain that it is possible to diagnose the origins of many diseases of internal organs by noticing to what part of the body the pain is referred. We have all learned from watching movies that sudden pain

in the left arm in the absence of an injury to the left arm means heart attack. Physicians know a much longer list of relations between areas of pain referral and diseased internal organs.

For instance, a kidney stone passing through the ureter will generate an excruciating pain that moves from the lower back to the inguinal region and the pubic area, even to the scrotum. The pain moves with the stone as it runs down the ureter, with the pain always referred to the surface of the body. Pain generated by cardiac ischemia can be felt in the chest, in the left shoulder and arm, in the tips of the left fingers, and even sometimes in the left side of the jaw. Inflammation of the gall bladder or an impacted gallstone can produce a pain felt at the tip of the right shoulder. The pain of appendicitis is due to the inflammation of the appendix on the right portion of the large intestine, yet the pain usually begins in the left side of the abdomen and slowly moves toward the center. These patterns of referred pain are very constant from patient to patient and are extremely useful tools for diagnosing the underlying disease. The area of referral is larger at the peak of the pain and gets smaller as the pain wanes. Referred pain is therefore a very dynamic phenomenon, immediately related to the originating cause but felt in areas of the body away from and sometimes remote from the diseased organ, which shows that the cause for the faulty localization is in the brain and not in the organ itself.

The explanation for referred pain is that, unlike pain from the skin, the muscles, and the joints that follows defined pathways within the spinal cord and the brain, visceral pain doesn't have a private highway of its own and has to hitch a ride on sensory pathways that carry information from the skin, the muscles, and the joints. This is called *convergence*, meaning that sensory nerves from internal organs converge in the brain on nerve cells that normally are driven by sensory nerves from the skin, the muscles, and the joints. The first place this convergence can occur is in the spinal cord, at the point where sensory nerves from the viscera and from the skin terminate. Those from the skin are organized in pathways that carry sensory information to the brain, where eventually they produce perceptions of well-localized sensations from the skin. Sensory nerves from the viscera are fewer in number (fewer than 10 percent of all sensory nerves come from the internal organs), are less well organized, and connect in a more diffuse way with nerve cells of the skin and muscle sensory pathways. Under normal circumstances, these pathways are activated by messages coming from the skin and the muscles. Throughout life we learn to identify these messages as sensa-

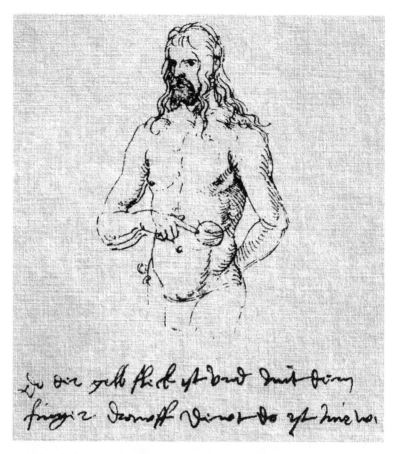

Figure 7.1
An example of pain referred to the surface of the body. This is a self-portrait of the German painter Albrecht Dürer (1471–1528) in which he wrote (in German) "There, where the yellow spot is located, and where I point my finger, there it hurts." Dürer drew this picture to show it to his physician and seek treatment for his pain, which was due to an unidentified disease of internal origin. This copy of the drawing appeared in the 1987 book *Classical German Contributions to Pain Research*. The original drawing is in the Kunsthalle in Bremen.

tions coming from the skin and the muscles. But one day, unexpectedly, our appendix is inflamed, or we have a kidney stone, or our heart nociceptors are activated by cardiac ischemia, and the signals generated end in the same pathways that have told us for years that when they are activated the sensation comes from the surface of the body. The brain receives these signals and makes the mistaken interpretation that the pain is coming from the skin and the muscles.

We know that the substrate for referred pain is a faulty localization because the area of referral remains constant even if we move our internal organs. In the case of organs such as the stomach or the intestine, this can be done, by taking deep breaths that will displace the contents of the abdomen a considerable distance. Referred pain from an inflamed gut will not move in the same way with the respiratory movement, which shows that the cause of the referral is in the brain's interpretation of the signal rather than in the inflamed organ itself. Another remarkable aspect of referred pain is that the area of referral can become more sensitive to pain—hyperalgesic—even though it is absolutely normal and the cause of the pain is far way. This also demonstrates that referred pain and referred hyperalgesia are brain-mediated phenomena, induced by convergence of visceral sensory nerves on skin and muscle sensory pathways.

Some people go through their entire lives without any of these alarm signals being activated. The brain has built a map of localization based on the origins of the most frequent sensory signals, including those that constantly come from the skin, the muscles, and the joints. It makes sense not to waste resources building private pathways for signals that may never occur. When something happens to our internal organs, an alarm is triggered that attracts our attention. It isn't particularly important that the localization be absolutely accurate. The anatomical pattern of convergence of somatic and visceral sensory nerves within the spinal cord will determine where in the surface of our bodies we will feel sensations when visceral nerves are activated. We know that sensory nerves from the heart converge on nerve cells that carry information from the left arm, those from the ureters converge on nerve cells that transmit information from the back and the groin, and so on.

Localization of Visceral Pain: A Diffuse Alarm System

The last two clinical properties of visceral pain that I mentioned at the beginning of this chapter are that it is very diffuse and badly localized and that it is always accompanied by exaggerated reactions, such as contracted muscles, changes in blood pressure, respiration, or sweating. These two properties highlight the diffuse nature of the pain, its poor localization, and the role of visceral pain as an unsophisticated yet effective alarm system.

A surprising fact about the signaling of visceral pain in our internal organs is that it is done by very few sensors—so few that the system is

incapable of accuracy and precise localization. Fewer than 10 percent of our sensory receptors are concerned with the signaling of visceral pain, yet the surface area of our internal organs is more than 200 times that of the skin, which receives 90 percent of all sensory nerves. If we consider these data, it is easy to understand why visceral pain is so diffuse and poorly localized relative to the much brighter and better-localized pain from the skin.

The mechanisms that the brain uses to process information from the internal organs are also different from those that deal with skin or muscle pain. Within the spinal cord and the brain, the very few sensory nerves connected to the viscera make many contacts with nerve cells, thereby generating a diffuse network of activated neurons that, although lacking in accuracy and in precise localization, can activate many regions of the brain and can maintain that activation for a long time. This organization functions very well as an alarm system. The activation of these few visceral sensors—our internal trip wires—produces a generalized excitation of sensory regions within the brain that leads to the perception of intense but poorly localized painful sensations. Modern techniques of brain imaging have demonstrated that injury or damage to internal organs capable of producing pain activates numerous brain areas concerned not only with the sensory perception of pain but also with emotional drives, endocrine regulation, control of movement, and cognition. It is a generalized and all-encompassing activation that tells us that something is wrong inside us and that something must be done about it. Interestingly, the same brain-imaging studies have also shown that visceral pain activates different brain regions in males than in females.

Functional Visceral Pain

Intuitively, we think that if we feel a pain in one leg, in one arm, or in our belly the cause of the pain must be in the leg, in the arm, or in the belly. However, pain perception is a brain function, and what we ultimately perceive is always a result of brain activity. Often a pain in a leg is due to an injury to the leg, but this is by no means an absolute rule. An alteration in the activity of the nerve cells in the brain that are concerned with sensory perceptions from the legs may result in a feeling of a painful sensation from the leg, even if there is nothing wrong in the leg itself. This is a very simple rule of the functions of our brain, yet for many people, including some members of the medical profession, this isn't immediately obvious. If a patient complains of a diffuse pain inside his

belly and physicians can't find anything wrong with his gut or his bladder, it is likely that the pain will be classified as psychogenic and the patient will be labeled a psychiatric case, which will make the life of the patient more miserable and will reduce the chances of recovery.

What I am describing here is a kind of pain known as *functional pain*. The word *functional* is used as an opposite to *organic*, which is the term used when an anatomical lesion of an organ or any other part of the body is evident. If there is a lesion that we can identify, it is labeled organic pain—evident and respectable. If there is no obvious damage anywhere, it is labeled functional pain—not so evident and definitely less respectable. It is only very recently that functional-pain syndromes have been identified as such and have gained recognition among some members of the medical profession. The stigma of the word *psychogenic* (usually meaning "not real") is still attached to patients suffering from functional-pain disorders.

An interesting aspect of functional-pain disorders is that many of them are characterized by pain felt in the inside of the body and often related to digestive or reproductive functions. Common functional-pain disorders include irritable bowel syndrome, interstitial cystitis, chronic pelvic pain, and functional dyspepsia. Other functional-pain syndromes not necessary associated with internal organs are fibromyalgia and chronic fatigue syndrome. Comorbidity (that is, presence of several forms of functional pain in the same patient) is very frequent, and many of the patients suffering from functional pain also suffer from social, economic, or psychological problems. This reinforces the preconception that the pain isn't real and there it must be due to some kind of psychological or psychiatric alteration.

Functional-pain disorders are more frequent in women, with prevalence rates as high as four times those in men. Some of these disorders are also associated with the female reproductive organs and are more prevalent in post-menopausal women, which has led to the belief that female hormones may be involved in the pathophysiology of functional pain. We know that changes in the levels of estrogen can cause profound alterations in pain perception, and that hormonal variations during the menstrual cycle can also influence the intensity of the symptoms of women suffering from chronic pelvic pain, interstitial cystitis, or irritable bowel syndrome. However, a direct association between hormonal alterations and these syndromes hasn't yet been established. Hormone-replacement therapy seems to be beneficial in reducing chronic pelvic pain and other functional-pain syndromes in post-menopausal women,

but whether this is due to a direct action of estrogen on the pain system or to a generalized improvement in the quality of life of these women isn't clear.

There are two potential mechanisms of functional pain. The first is that there is indeed a problem at the level of the peripheral organ—the gut, the bladder, or the uterus—but that it isn't detectable with standard diagnostic tools. A number of such small alterations have been found in the bladders of patients with interstitial cystitis, and there is evidence of some kind of subtle chronic inflammatory process in patients with irritable bowel syndrome. But these alterations could be due to changes in the functioning of internal organs as a consequence of the chronic pain felt by the patients. We may be facing a chicken-and-egg situation that is also applicable to the psychological comorbidity shown by these patients. On the one hand, a life of chronic pain may induce alterations in internal organs that eventually produce small lesions and social and psychological disturbances. On the other hand, these small lesions or these psychological disturbances may be the cause of the chronic pain. We still don't know what is the sequence of events in these patients.

The second interpretation is based on current knowledge about sensitization of pain pathways. We know that the peripheral nerve sensors in internal organs and the entire pain pathway from the organs to the spinal cord and the brain can become more excitable when repeatedly activated. We believe that this is the mechanism of *hyperalgesia*, the increased sensitivity to pain that often occurs after a lesion of or damage to the skin or the internal organs. Therefore, a possible mechanism of functional pain is that such hyperexcitability of the visceral-pain pathway develops without a peripheral cause or is maintained beyond the duration of a peripheral stimulus. A number of molecular targets have been identified in visceral sensory nerves and in brain cells in the pain pathway capable of maintaining the excitability of the pathway beyond the duration of the originating stimulus. It is possible that a relatively minor event in the gut, the bladder, or the reproductive organs, coupled with an unpleasant personal experience could trigger an enhanced sensitivity of the visceral-pain pathway that remains for years after the originating event.

Functional-pain disorders are puzzling. It is possible that they are triggered by small and difficult-to-detect alterations in internal organs. We know that some reproductive hormones can influence the magnitude of these pain disorders. It is also likely that a relatively minor life event could transform a small alteration of an internal organ into a chronic-pain process. And it is clear that visceral-pain pathways can

show long-lasting enhancements of excitability that account for increased sensitivity to pain from internal organs in the absence of a major injury or disease to the organ. These disorders have been recently recognized as real pain syndromes, which is the first step toward finding a mechanism and eventually a cure for them.

Treating Visceral Pain

When faced with treating a patient with visceral pain, we have two not very satisfactory options: either use analgesics that weren't specifically developed to treat visceral pain or treat the originating disease and hope that the pain will go away. Unfortunately, there are very few specific treatments for the pain of visceral disease and even fewer for functional forms of pain.

Classical analgesics attenuate pain perception in general (as the opiates do) or reduce inflammatory reactions (as aspirin and ibuprofen do). We still use many of these analgesics in a non-specific way to deal with all forms of pain. No currently available analgesics are aimed at reducing pain of internal origin. Some of the more powerful analgesics, including the opiates, are counter-indicated in cases of visceral disease, as opiates induce contractions of the smooth muscle in the walls of the internal organs and make the pain from these organs even worse. Because of the close relation between the activities of internal organs and the sensations that originate from them, a conventional way to treat visceral pain has been to reduce the activity of the organ in question. This is the rationale for the use of drugs that reduce the muscle tone of the gut, the ureter, or the bladder and drugs decrease gastrointestinal secretions. The basic idea is that by reducing the motor and secretary activity of an organ we also reduce the chances of activation of the sensors that signal pain from the organ. But these compounds don't have analgesic activity by themselves; for this reason, reducing the activity of the organ will have little effect on the perception of pain if the sensory nerves are sensitized or hyperactive.

A patient with internal pain due to a well-established pathology will obviously see a specialist on that pathology—for example, a cardiologist, a gastroenterologist, an urologist, or a gynecologist. Most such specialists concentrate on the underlying condition and regard the pain only as a by-product of the disease that will go away once the patient is cured. Many medical specialists don't see pain as a disease in its own right—as something that must be treated independently of the originating disease.

This is why patients suffering from functional-pain syndromes such as irritable bowel syndrome or interstitial cystitis have had difficulty getting their conditions recognized as genuine. Since it is often difficult or even impossible to find an organic cause in their guts or bladders for their symptoms, they are easily labeled hysterical, hypochondriacal, or psychologically disturbed.

Yet, as was discussed earlier in this chapter, many patients with functional-pain disorders also show psycho-social morbidity. Though it isn't easy to tell which of these is causing the other, it is nevertheless a fact that many such patients benefit from psychological counseling or from learning to accept their pain and how to live with it. The recently developed drugs indicated for functional-pain syndromes act within the brain and are aimed at modifying behavior by reducing anxiety, eliminate depressive thoughts, and improve the quality of life. These behavioral changes can reduce the influence of pain on a patient's life.

8　A Mere Curse: Neuropathic Pain

I will open this chapter with a real story that dramatically illustrates the appalling curse of neuropathic pain. A young English nurse was on vacation in Turkey. She boarded a very overcrowded public bus and had to stand in the aisle, squeezed among dozens of travelers, trying to keep her balance by holding on to a bar above her head very tightly. The bus was traveling at high speed on a bumpy and twisty road. It toppled over and tumbled, and its roof broke apart, carrying with it the bar that our nurse was grabbing. Her arm, with the hand still holding on to the bar, was torn from her body. When I met her, a few years after the crash, the wounds had long healed but she was able to describe very vividly how she saw, as in a slow-motion movie, the roof of the bus fly away, and with it her arm. The most astonishing thing is that at the time of the accident, overwhelmed by panic at what was happening around her, she felt no pain. After a few days in a hospital, she was discharged and returned home. And then the problems began. First she began feeling as if her lost arm was still there—a phantom limb. She could feel the missing arm, the missing hand, and the missing fingers. But it wasn't a normal arm, for the feelings weren't proportional to the size of the original limb. The hand seemed to be too close to her shoulder, as if the arm were very short. This so-called telescoping is very frequent among amputees. The phantom limb also feels itchy, tingly, or prickly. These sensations, which aren't painful, are felt by all amputees, but a smaller group of patients—among them our nurse—experience painful sensations from the phantom limb.

The pain begins months or even years after an amputation and progresses from very occasional to almost constant. For our nurse, the sensations were those that one would normally associate with an arm being twisted and torn. She was in fact reliving her accident, which at the time was painless but which now produced a very real pain linked to the trauma. The phantom arm not only seemed to be an integral part of her

body; it also felt compressed, pulled, and torn. She was constantly having her arm torn away time after time, and on each occasion she would feel the expected pain.

These painful sensations are so bizarre that the sufferers think they must be going crazy. There are some treatments that we can prescribe for these patients, from drugs to exercises to playing with mirrors, but the most important thing is to reassure them that they aren't imagining their pain or losing their mind. Phantom-limb pain is a very real pain—a kind of *neuropathic* pain. The painful sensations have no relationship with a real injury or are felt in parts of the body that are now missing. There is no longer a reason for the pain, no explanation that can make sense, no protective justification. Neuropathic pain is pain in the absence of logic, often without any trigger, present all the time or in waves. It is plainly abnormal. There is nothing useful about it. It is always an expression of a damaged nervous system. It may be caused by a major trauma (e.g. an amputation), or by an injury as minor as a sprained ankle, or by a tiny lesion within the brain. There are numerous forms of neuropathic pain, but in all cases the pain has no proportional relationship with an external cause, appears without an apparent reason, is triggered by stimuli that normally aren't painful, and ruins the patient's life.

Neuropathic Pain: What's in a Name?

Scientists and physicians are fond of definitions, classification, and the naming of the parts. We think that defining a process and classifying its components leads to understanding. We invent new words to qualify what we don't know and believe that by using these words we advance our knowledge. And, unfortunately, we get tangled in discussions about the meanings of these words without realizing that we invented them in the first place because we didn't fully understand the process we wanted to define.

That brings us to the definition of neuropathic pain. Not long ago, all forms of pain were regarded as products of a single process. Therefore, a unique mechanism—a pain pathway or a pattern of nerve impulses— was thought to explain everything from the pain of a simple injury to that of a phantom limb. It is hard to believe that only in the last few decades was a general agreement reached among pain scientists and physicians that there are many kinds of pain and therefore many different pain mechanisms. That agreement followed the realization that some forms of pain (e.g. the pain of an acute injury or an inflammation) were

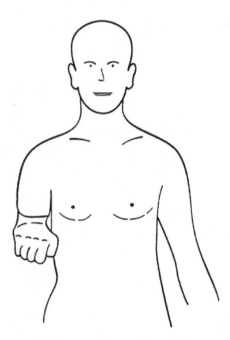

Figure 8.1
A schematic drawing of an amputee showing where he feels the missing right arm. The phantom hand gradually approaches the residual limb and eventually becomes located inside the stump. From L. Nikolajsen and T. S. Jensen, "Phantom limb pain," *British Journal of Anaesthesia* 87 (2001): 107–116.

normal and others (e.g. phantom-limb pain or postherpetic neuralgia) were abnormal. Abnormal pains were grouped under the term *neuro-pathic* to indicate that they are caused by a pathological nervous system. In contrast, the word *nociceptive*, referring to the perception of a noxious event, was used to qualify normal pain, a sensation that everyone feels after an injury.

The logical conclusion is that the mechanisms of normal (nociceptive) pain and those of abnormal (neuropathic) pain may be different, and that therefore an accurate identification of nociceptive and neuropathic pain was crucial for the separation of the two forms of pain and for the development of suitable therapeutic strategies. How do we distinguish neuropathic from nociceptive pain? Do we have clear and accurate definitions?

The International Association for the Study of Pain, which has an active taxonomy group dedicated to putting forward definitions for pain-related terms, first defined neuropathic pain as "pain initiated or

caused by a primary lesion or dysfunction of the nervous system" and more recently changed it to "pain caused by a lesion or disease of the somatosensory nervous system." The changes introduced in the latest definition have been the subject of considerable discussion, as they are not as minor as they would initially appear. Both definitions suggest that neuropathic pain is caused by a damaged nervous system, and that abnormal pain appears when the nervous system isn't working properly. The differences between the two definitions lie in the replacement of the word *dysfunction* by *disease* and in the narrowing of the focus from the entire nervous system to the *somatosensory* nervous system as the originator of the pain.

The first change is a matter of precision. *Dysfunction* is a word that sounds respectable in principle, but when examined in detail it doesn't define a well-shaped concept. How can we detect and measure a dysfunction? What is a dysfunction, anyway? The new definition puts the emphasis on demonstrable and measurable alterations of neural function: a lesion, a disease. But in doing so it also tests our medical knowledge and leaves out of the neuropathic pain group those conditions for which, at present, we are not able to identify a specific lesion or disease. And the new definition leaves out some very well known and prevalent forms of what was traditionally thought to be neuropathic pain—hence the intense debate triggered by the new meaning of neuropathic pain. The problems of finding a lesion or a disease at the origin of some types of neuropathic pain will be discussed later in the chapter, but it is relevant to remark here that, in order for a pain to be considered neuropathic, an identifiable lesion of the nervous system is now required. And this also means that the list of neuropathic pain conditions remains open to future advances in medical knowledge.

The second change focuses on the somatosensory nervous system, a component of the nervous system that deals with sensory information from the body's exterior and interior (including muscles and internal organs but excluding those senses that signal external events, such as vision or hearing). Also excluded form the somatosensory system are brain functions such as control of movement or mental activity. This restriction imposes a compartmentalized vision of the brain and goes against the idea of the pain experience being the overall result of activity in many brain areas. It is, in fact, very difficult to break up the nervous system into parcels and compartments; we do it to facilitate our limited understanding, but the brain doesn't recognize borders and boundaries within itself and doesn't know what the somatosensory

system is. Where are the limits of the somatosensory nervous system? Where does it begin and where does it end? Isn't it possible to have pain as a consequence of lesions of brain areas concerned with emotions or rational thoughts?

The current definition of neuropathic pain demands the identification of a lesion or a disease, which, whatever its boundaries are, must be restricted to the somatosensory nervous system. The diagnostic process requires careful analysis of the pain in search of the lesion and its locus. However, even though many neuropathic pain conditions share common symptoms (e.g., spontaneous pain, burning pain, touch-evoked pain, or feelings of extreme cold), this doesn't indicate common mechanisms, and these symptoms don't necessarily lead to the diagnosis of an identifiable disease. Also, it is more accurate to talk about neuropathic *pains* (plural) caused by very different diseases than about a single kind of neuropathic pain. These are the reasons why further classification of neuropathic pain conditions is based not on their symptoms or their mechanisms but on whether the originating neural lesion is located in the peripheral nervous system (the nerves that run through our limbs and bodies) or in the spinal cord and the brain (the central nervous system itself). Let us look at these enigmatic and dreadful pain conditions by following this peripheral-versus-central approach.

Lessons of War

One of the most influential books in the study of neuropathic pain was a direct result of the American Civil War. It was written by Silas Weir Mitchell, a Philadelphia neurologist born into a family of several generations of physicians. The book, titled *Injuries of Nerves and Their Consequences* and published in 1872, was based on a clinical study of soldiers injured during the Civil War that Mitchell, in collaboration with several other physicians, first published in 1864 as *Gunshot Wounds and Other Injuries of Nerves*. These books contain detailed observations of the pain symptoms experienced by soldiers who sustained gunshot injuries and include the first modern descriptions of peripheral neuropathic pain. They are also written in a very readable style. (Mitchell was an accomplished author who later in his life wrote novels and poetry.)

Mitchell's patients, including nearly 100 soldiers who had received gunshot wounds in various battles, had nerve injuries of many kinds and to virtually every major nerve of the body. The nerve injuries varied from patient to patient; however, all the patients had lesions, which ranged

from bruising to contusion or inflammation to partial or complete section of major nerves. Most of the wounds were to the limbs and neck and affected the larger nerves that run through the arms and legs. Regardless of the type of injury or the part of the body that had been damaged, there were common symptoms and signs that led Mitchell to label the pain caused by a traumatic nerve injury *causalgia*, a word made up from the Greek words for "burning" and "pain."

One of Mitchell's observations was that about one-third of the soldiers didn't feel any pain at the time of injury and weren't aware of having been shot until they saw their blood or fell to the ground with a broken or paralyzed leg. These were soldiers who had been shot while engaged in active combat. Those who felt pain (the other two-thirds) hadn't been fighting when they were injured. This observation illustrates very well that pain perception can be eliminated by intense stress, a topic that will be discussed in more detail in the next chapter.

The pain caused by the nerve injuries had several phases. Initially there was little sensation in the area of innervation, or even complete anesthesia if the nerve had been severed. But then, after a period of time that could be as long as weeks or months, a different kind of pain appeared in the previously insensitive portion of the skin that was innervated by the damaged nerve. The pain was described as burning, as if the skin was on fire or a red-hot iron was being pushed through the limb. Pain could be triggered by the slightest stimulus, such as a brief touch or a gentle stroking of the skin, but it could also be present all the time, without the need for a stimulus, a constant burning sensation through the affected limb whose intensity was so great that it became overpowering to the point of changing the life of the patient. Mitchell tells us that these veterans looked thin, nervous, and worn out, that they were sleeping badly because of the pain, and that the disease had ruined their lives. One former sergeant was described as having gone from being a man of "kindly temper" to being "morose and melancholy."

And that isn't all. The nerve injury also produces *trophic* changes— structural alterations of the skin, muscles, and joints of the territory innervated by the damaged nerve. The skin over the limb looks glossy, red, shiny, and tight. Muscles are contracted, fixing fingers or toes in extreme positions. Hair falls out, and the nails are overgrown, clubbed, and yellow. The damaged limb also shows changes in sweating, sometimes being damp and sometimes dry for no obvious reason. When x-ray techniques were introduced, it was also noticed that the bones of the affected limb were atrophying (that is, losing their strength). Many of the

patients arrived clutching their injured limbs, even months or years after the original wound, the arms or legs looking wasted and the sufferer protecting the limb from being touched or keeping it wet all the time as to reduce the burning sensation. Mitchell describes the disease dramatically: "Perhaps few persons who are not physicians can realize the influence which long-continued and unendurable pain may have on both body and mind. Under such torments the temper changes, the most amiable grow irritable, the bravest soldier becomes a coward, and the strongest man is scarcely less nervous than the most hysterical girl. Perhaps nothing can better illustrate the extent to which these statements may be true than the cases of burning pain, or, as I prefer to term it, Causalgia, the most terrible of all tortures which a nerve wound may inflict."

Mitchell's study of the gunshot wounds of Civil War veterans first established the symptoms and characteristics of *causalgia*, but there are many other alterations of peripheral nerves that lead to similar conditions. Any traumatic nerve injury can generate the disease, including damage to nerves during surgical operations. A proportion of patients undergoing surgery may end up with a painful neuropathy even after relatively minor operations, such as plastic surgery or repair of an inguinal hernia. General diseases such as diabetes or a herpes infection can also produce peripheral nerve damage, leading to painful conditions similar to causalgia. In the case of diabetes, the high levels of glucose cause damage to a variety of peripheral nerves—diabetic neuropathy— that in turn can produce pain. Sometimes this happens after many years. Some patients develop post-herpetic neuralgia (pain after a herpes infection), with symptoms that include the constant burning sensation and the trophic changes characteristic of causalgia. Nerve damage can also be caused by toxic products, including alcohol and some anti-cancer drugs, and patients to whom this happens may also develop painful neuropathies. Thus, there is a wide range of conditions that can cause nerve damage and lead to peripheral neuropathic pain.

The most enigmatic aspect of this kind of pain is the variability of its prevalence among the various groups of patients. Traumatic nerve injuries generate chronic pain in about 5–15 percent of patients. The proportion is higher among soldiers wounded in combat, some statistics showing percentages as high as 40. Post-surgical chronic pain can develop in about 10 percent of patients. Painful diabetic neuropathy occurs in about 15 percent of long-term diabetics and post-herpetic neuralgia in less than 10 percent of patients. These are all relatively low figures. They show that

only a small proportion of patients develop chronic burning pain after a peripheral neuropathy.

Why is that some people develop chronic pain and others don't after similar traumas and diseases? Unfortunately, we don't know. In the next chapter we will examine factors such as stress, genetic background, and sex. We know that there are social and economic factors, but we don't know how they come into play. What is it that generates chronic pain in some people but not in others after very similar injures and diseases? This is one of the most challenging questions we face in our search for knowledge about pain mechanisms.

And there is another problem. Some people develop symptoms that resemble those of causalgia, including excruciating chronic pain, in the absence of a nerve injury or after very minor trauma. A patient will go to a physician complaining of burning pain in an arm or a leg or of "electric shock" pain, sometimes accompanied by trophic alterations of hair and nail growth, skin redness, and sweating. The patient believes that these symptoms are caused by a minor injury (perhaps a twisted ankle or a sprained wrist), but after extensive exploration no significant nerve damage can be found. In the late 1940s a new term was coined to describe this condition: *reflex sympathetic dystrophy* (RSD). The rationale for this name was that the disease was some kind of exaggerated reflex to a minor injury, and that it was mediated by the sympathetic nervous system (the component of peripheral nerves that is in charge of controlling blood flow, sweating, and other such functions). The name stuck even though there was never any evidence that this was a reflex reaction, that it was mediated by the sympathetic nervous system, or that the prime symptom was a degenerative disease.

About 20 years ago, trying to bring some order to this messy field, a group of experts proposed that all causalgia-like conditions be put under the umbrella of a new name, *Complex Regional Pain Syndrome* (CRPS), and further subdivided the diseases of this group into CRPS-type I (for those with no major apparent cause, such as the old RSD) and CRPS-type II (for those with obvious evidence of nerve damage, such as causalgia). Though this sorting exercise helped experts to catalog these diseases, it also generated two very serious problems with CRPS-type I, one mechanistic and the other a consequence of human nature.

The mechanistic problem is that we now have a set of diseases, which we label CRPS-type I, whose diagnostic criteria require the lack of any possible explanation, which makes them not amenable to the scientific method. If a disease is defined by not being produced by an identifiable

cause, it is technically impossible to approach it scientifically. Moreover, the current definition of neuropathic pain, which requires that the pain be caused by a lesion or a disease of the nervous system, wouldn't apply to these conditions, thus generating the paradox that one subclass of CRPS is neuropathic and the other is not. For scientists trying to unravel the mechanisms of pain, it is very disappointing to know that a major pain disease can be defined only by our inability to find a cause. In other words, if you find a nerve lesion in a patient, that patient no longer can have that particular disease.

The second problem is even trickier. Pain is subjective and can't be accurately measured independently of the patients' reports. The objective signs of CRPS-type I, among them skin changes and muscle contractures, aren't always necessary to establish a diagnosis and in some cases can be induced by immobility or forced postures. Since the symptoms are subjective and the diagnostic criteria include not finding an objective lesion, the door is opened to patients who express psychiatric symptoms or, even worse, to malingerers. And there is evidence that among the patients diagnosed with CRPS-type I there are some psychiatric cases and malingerers. This is not to say that this condition doesn't exist, but we must be honest with ourselves and consider alternative options. In the long run, that will be the best service we can offer to patients whose symptoms are indeed produced by an objective lesion of their peripheral nerves.

Damage at Command and Control

Another real and dramatic story of a patient who developed neuropathic pain involves a 40-year-old married man with four children—a solid, dependable, hard-working person who managed a shopping center. He worked long hours but still found time to look after his children and enjoy his family. One day, out of the blue, his life changed forever. While working at the shopping center, he suddenly felt an intense headache. The pain was so strong that he felt that he was about to pass out. People around him noticed that this was more than a minor headache and called an ambulance. By then, our man began to feel as if cold water was being poured over about half of his body. But there was no water anywhere. This made him even more anxious, since he couldn't understand what was going on. Half of his body felt wet and cold, but his colleagues were telling him that he wasn't cold and that he was imagining things. After he was rushed to a hospital, the physicians immediately suspected what

was going on and put him through a brain scanner. The instant diagnosis was that he had just suffered a very small localized brain hemorrhage—a stroke.

The scan showed that inside the man's brain there was a small hemangioma—an abnormal growth of tangled blood vessels that, when it happens in the skin, produces a distinctive purple red patch. His very small hemangioma was deep inside his brain, close to the thalamus (the brain's main sensory nucleus). Because the tangled blood vessels aren't very strong and tend to break, such benign growths can go unnoticed for years except when they occur inside the vital part of an organ. Our man's hemangioma had a broken blood vessel that produced a small hemorrhage deep inside the brain; that explained the intense headache. He was operated on immediately. The bleeding was stopped and the hemangioma was dealt with, but by then some parts of the thalamus had suffered permanent damage caused by compression and a lack of blood.

The man recovered, left the hospital, went back to work, and tried to return to a normal life. He still works hard, looks after his family, and exercises every day, but now he has a constant feeling of intense cold over half of his body, from the toes to the leg to the abdomen and thorax to the upper arm and neck. He feels as if he is constantly half-immersed in ice-cold water, a feeling that isn't changed by wearing or not wearing clothes or by the outside temperature (hot or cold) and isn't related to the actual temperature of his skin. The cold is so intense and so constant that it is very painful. It doesn't stop at night, and he hardly sleeps. He is anxious at times and depressed at other times. Having been a pillar of society, the sort of man who will not miss a day's work for any reason, and hence a little intolerant of other peoples' weaknesses, he now worries that his colleagues may not believe him and that they may think he is making these things up. He is tortured by the thought that he may be going crazy. Above all, he wonders what is wrong with him and why he is now in such appalling state.

The diagnosis for this patient is *central post-stroke pain* (formerly known as *thalamic syndrome*), a particularly nasty kind of neuropathic pain caused by lesions of the main sensory pathway inside the brain that carries pain and temperature signals. His life has been completely changed forever. His physician can do little for him other than prescribe analgesics (which may not work very well) and other medications that will help him through his bouts of anxiety and depression. His physician

will recommend, however, that he go to a psychologist who will help him learn to adapt to and live with his pain. This patient is another victim of central neuropathic pain.

Most of the lesions that cause central neuropathic pain are consequences of vascular problems within the brain—either blood clots or hemorrhages. Such lesions can occur anywhere in the brain, but when they affect the regions that deal with pain signals they produce bizarre symptoms, including vivid sensory hallucinations of pain and temperature. The sensations are very real, and the patients suffer considerably, but there is nothing in their bodies that remotely explains what they feel. All these sensations are products of a sick brain. Because of the relationship between vascular diseases and central neuropathic pain, these syndromes are more common among older people, adding the misery of constant pain to their other ailments. Occasionally they can happen in younger patients, such as the man mentioned above, as a result of vascular tumors or caused by diseases and events that produce very high blood pressure. Degenerative diseases of the central nervous system, such as multiple sclerosis, can also cause central neuropathic pain, as can brain tumors and malformations. The results are always the same: sensory hallucinations (including a relentless feeling of pain projected to an otherwise normal part of the body) and resistance to most common analgesics.

Central neuropathic pain appears when a lesion within the central nervous system affects the main pathways and centers that carry information about the sensory component of pain. This is why the most frequent kind is when the damage affects the thalamus (the brain's main sensory nucleus), and why this disease was originally called *thalamic syndrome*. We now know that similar symptoms can also appear after lesions of other parts of the pain pathway; hence the widening of the term. In all cases the main symptoms are sensory—that is, directly related to the basic quality of pain. The patients feel constant and intense pain, usually associated with a temperature element. (Pain and temperature signals travel together in the brain.) Sometimes the sensations are sharp; sometimes they feel like prickle or itch or tingling. The pain is constant and spontaneous but can be made worse by mild stimuli applied to the region of the skin where the pain is projected. Because there is no obvious cause for their bizarre sensations, not only do the patients suffer; they also tend to think they are imagining things and may be losing their minds. But the explanation is relatively simple. What has happened is

that the machine that we have for sensing, processing, and experiencing pain inside our brain has broken down.

A Broken Machine

The nurse with phantom-limb pain, the soldiers Silas Weir Mitchell studied, and the man with the brain hemorrhage are very different clinical cases. However, they all have one common feature that makes them all neuropathic-pain patients: their nervous systems aren't working properly. Something has broken down inside the brain. And if the control machine is faulty, weird experiences can happen.

There are many mechanisms of neuropathic pain, which are likely to differ from disease to disease and even from patient to patient. This is characteristic of a set of diseases that are produced by pathological changes in the nervous system; the individual symptoms depend on the extent and the nature of the lesion generated by the specific pathology. The nerve damage produced by long-term diabetes is different from that caused by a herpes infection or that caused by a traumatic lesion of a single nerve. Equally, the amount of brain tissue damaged after a hemorrhage or a degenerative lesion is variable and unique for each patient. But we have some knowledge of what happens in the peripheral and the central nervous system when damage occurs, and from this knowledge we can infer some basic mechanisms that may be responsible for the neuropathic pain we see in patients.

A big caveat is called for here: Most of what we have learned about neural damage comes from laboratory studies, in which researchers try to reproduce in experimental animals, in tissues, or in individual cells the lesions and the pathologies that physicians see in patients. Yet animal models only approximate the clinical conditions. By their very nature, laboratory lesions are controlled and accurate, in contrast to whatever causes most clinically relevant pain syndromes. Assessing neuropathic pain in laboratory animals is even harder than assessing normal pain, as we can't measure abnormal sensory perceptions or changes in the features of a pain experience in an animal. For obvious ethical reasons, laboratory tests tend to be brief and restricted, which is also contrary to the length and the intensity of the expression of most neuropathic pain conditions in humans. Therefore, our knowledge of the mechanisms of neuropathic pain focuses mainly on basic processes, among them changes in neuronal excitability or in synaptic plasticity. What we know best is what happens to individual nerves and neurons when they are

damaged by trauma, or by anything else. But how this damage leads to the complex and abnormal sensory experiences that we see in patients is still unknown.

Most people would think that damaging or cutting a peripheral nerve would render the area of distribution of that nerve insensitive. Though this is true in the earlier phases of a nerve lesion, the long-term effects are almost the opposite. Damaged nerves become hyperexcitable; they generate nerve signals or action potentials spontaneously and at high frequencies, and they become an uncontrolled source of nerve activity, which they project toward the brain. We believe that this is the reason for the bizarre sensations reported by people with peripheral nerve damage, ranging from tingling or buzzing to spontaneous pain. The increased activity that arises from a nerve injury, known in the trade as *ectopic activity*, leads to experiences felt in the part of the body innervated by the damaged nerve even though the signals are now generated within the nerve itself. Damaged nerves also become sensitive to touch or tapping, so normal movements of the limb add to the generation of abnormal signals and thus to pain.

The impulses generated at a point of nerve injury can also travel toward the skin, the muscles, or the joints, where they can release inflammatory compounds that contribute to the sensitization of the pain sensors (nociceptors). Nerve damage also affects the sympathetic nerves that control blood flow, sweating, and other structural elements of the skin, which would explain the trophic alterations seen after peripheral nerve damage or neuropathy. These skin reactions can also be normal consequences of the increased nerve activity induced at the point of damage. The central nervous system reacts to the abnormal sensory barrage as if the skin had been injured even though the lesion is of the nerves and not of the skin.

A neuropathic pain condition that begins with a peripheral nerve injury evokes a pain experience that is always a result of the involvement of the central nervous system. There are indeed many changes that happen in a peripheral nerve when it is damaged, but it is the reaction of the brain to these changes that eventually generates the neuropathic pain experience. Silas Weir Mitchell had already noted that "we have some doubt as to whether this form of pain [i.e., causalgia] ever originates at the moment of the wounding" and that "the burning arises later, almost always during the healing of the wound." This very accurate observation implies a reactive change of the central nervous system to the peripheral nerve injury. In turn, the abnormal activity generated

by a nerve lesion triggers changes within the brain that cause neuropathic pain. This seems to be the case in diabetic neuropathy, in postherpetic neuralgia (in which the nerve lesion is limited to some types of nerve fiber and the resulting imbalance of activity generates first abnormal sensations and then pain), and in deafferentation pain (a kind of neuropathic pain caused by a lack of sensory input from an area of the body due to nerve damage). The imbalance between the signals generated from different body regions leads to abnormal sensations, including pain.

Under normal circumstances, the brain is constantly bombarded with sensory signals from external and internal sensors; it deals with these sensory barrages by applying a substantial amount of inhibition to them, letting through only those signals that are useful for an appropriate reaction at any moment. We think that an important component of neuropathic pain is a lifting of this brain inhibition due either to a lesion of the brain itself (as in central neuropathic pain) or to the barrage of abnormal impulses generated by nerve damage in a peripheral neuropathy. This is the process known as *disinhibition*. We believe it plays an important role in the generation of chronic-pain states, particularly those that produce neuropathic pain.

Disinhibition contributes to enhanced brain activity that can eventually become explosive, a form of epilepsy. Neuropathic-pain patients describe their pain as explosive and overpowering. The fact that antiepileptic drugs are very useful in the treatment of neuropathic pain suggests that the two diseases have common features. The consequences of disinhibition include enhanced activity of neurons in the brain, sensitization of pain pathways, and general increases in the excitability of the cells that transmit pain signals. In addition, the increased activity that results from disinhibition can stimulate synaptic plasticity or even structural changes of the brain, especially when the painful process becomes chronic. We know that persistent pain can change the structure of the brain, and the combination of increased neural activity and the plasticity induced by the neural lesions offers a possible explanation for these structural changes.

There are some neuropathic pain conditions (phantom-limb pain is a very good example) whose mechanisms have both peripheral and central components. An amputation always results in the severing of major nerves, and those nerves will be damaged even more if the amputation is traumatic rather than surgical . The ends of severed nerves develop a small growth area, know as a *neuroma*, that becomes extremely sensitive

to touch and to local inflammatory mediators. Because the brain interprets the signals coming from a neuroma as originating from the territory that the nerve used to innervate, the sensations are felt in the limb that is no longer there. And because the signals from the neuroma don't follow the normal pattern of activity that they had when they were generated by the intact limb, the sensations are bizarre and abnormal. Patients with phantom-limb pain often feel sensations in their missing limbs associated with other sensory perceptions or with certain behaviors, which shows that the brain integrates convergent sensory inputs into a global experience. In other patients, a pain experience from another part of the body can trigger a sensation of phantom-limb pain. There are reports of long-term amputees suddenly feeling pain in their missing limbs when suffering from angina or a duodenal ulcer. Phantom limbs can also be felt in awkward or extreme positions or in the position that the limb had when it was injured, as it was the case with the nurse mentioned at the beginning of this chapter. Even though signals are initially generated at the amputation site by the damaged nerves, it is the brain that ultimately produces the sensory experience that the patients feel.

Our knowledge of the mechanisms of neuropathic pain has advanced, but many important questions remain. It is puzzling that only a minority of people who suffer nerve damage, amputations, metabolic or degenerative diseases of their nerves, or even brain damage after a stroke develop neuropathic pain. Lacking an explanation for this, we blame external elements (including social and economic ones), or internal factors (including genetic ones), or even the age of the patient.

A strange feature of the neuropathic pain induced by nerve damage is that it occurs only when the injury affects some nerves but not others. It appears most often after lesions of the larger and longer nerves of the limbs, sometimes in the nerves of the face and neck, and rarely after injury of internal nerves. The teeth seem to be impervious to neuropathic pain; thousands of them are extracted every day around the world by a process that includes the tearing of nerves. Endodontic therapy (commonly known as a root-canal operation) is an everyday dental procedure that includes mashing the nerves inside a tooth, yet neuropathic pain of dental origin is extremely rare and almost never related to extractions or root-canal operations. We have no idea what makes a nerve more prone to triggering neuropathic pain after an injury.

And then there are the enigmatic conditions (CRPS-type I) for which no neural lesion is found. Whether or not we catalog them as

neuropathic, the fact remains that a whole set of pain-related symptoms, akin to those of causalgia or peripheral nerve injury, appear in patients who have no obvious lesion. Fibromyalgia, classified as a functional-pain syndrome, also falls into this category. Are these expressions of a more general disease of the brain? Are they psychiatric disorders? Is there an organic cause for them that remains to be identified? At present we have no definite answers.

9 Sex, Genes, and Stress: Pain Modulation

During World War II, as the Allied armies pushed northward through Italy, they met stiff resistance from German troops. The Allied High Command decided to outflank them with a landing on the beaches of Anzio, on Italy's west coast. The landing was a bloody operation, with many casualties on both sides. Although it was eventually successful for the Allies, the Germans managed to slow down the advance of the Allied troops for several months. Among the American medics at Anzio was a remarkable physician named Henry Beecher, a Harvard graduate from Kansas who specialized in anesthesiology. Beecher was one of the medical officers who sorted out the wounded soldiers and sent them from the front lines to hospitals in the rear. During that process, he decided to conduct some research by asking soldiers if they were in pain, how much pain they felt, and if they wanted any pain medication. He tabulated the answers carefully. Some years later, when the war was over and he was back in Boston working as an anesthesiologist at Massachusetts General Hospital, Beecher asked the same questions of a group of young patients who had just been through surgery, then compared their answers with the data he had collected from the soldiers. When the results were published, Beecher's observations from the Anzio beachhead entered the hall of fame of pain research.

The essential piece of data was that most of the injured soldiers, including many with extensive wounds, reported no pain at the time of their injury and didn't ask for pain medication. Beecher observed that many of them were in a highly excited state, and that although they were very much aware of their wounds only a minority reported pain. In contrast, the majority of the civilian surgical patients at the hospital, in a completely different setting, reported considerable pain and requested painkillers, even when their surgeries were less extensive (and obviously far better controlled) than the soldiers' injuries.

Beecher's explanation was that the wounded soldiers were glad to be alive and were aware that their injuries meant a period of recovery in a safe place and perhaps even discharge from the Army, and that this exultant emotional state reduced or even eliminated the pain. On the other hand, the surgical patients were worried about the consequences of the surgery, whether the operation had been successful, and how long it would take for them to recover, and this worrying made their pain worse. Beecher concluded that the emotional component of a pain experience is so powerful that the same injury can produce different amounts of pain depending on factors such as stress, sex, ethnicity, age, anxiety, expectation, suggestion, and even the weather.

Some years ago I read an article, written in 1939, in which the British physiologist J. B. S. Haldane described graphically how emotional and rational factors modulate the symptoms of disease. He wrote: "The commonest cause of gastritis, that is to say, an inflamed and irritable stomach, is worry and anxiety. I had it for fifteen years until I read Lenin and other writers who showed me what was wrong with our society and how to cure it. Since then I have needed no magnesia. But these pains may be due to gastric ulcer or even cancer. So, it is better to consult a doctor, even though he will probably recommend magnesia." Today it is hard to imagine that anyone would find Lenin's writings a helpful therapy for gastric ulcers. Yet the underlying sentiment still holds. Pain and disease can be powerfully influenced by our emotions and beliefs.

We tend to think that emotions are primeval reactions and that a more developed and rational brain, such as ours, has tamed and controlled them. This is a very simplistic view, especially when we reflect on how our emotions influence pain. We have already seen that a full pain experience has sensory, emotional, and cognitive elements, and we are pretty sure that these three components aren't organized in a hierarchical way, with one of them controlling another, but in a more cooperative way, with emotions, sensations, and rational thoughts interacting to generate the final pain experience. This interpretation is more in line with our knowledge of how the brain processes pain-related signals and better illustrates the extensive interaction that takes place among the three components of a pain experience.

A corollary of this interpretation is that sensory dysfunctions and maladaptive emotional reactions can lead to abnormal pain perceptions such as those characteristic of neuropathic pain. Not only may abnormal pains be due to a damaged brain mechanism; they may also be a conse-

quence of failing to modulate a pain experience appropriately. The evidence shows that the perception of pain is strongly influenced by many external and internal factors and not just by the magnitude of an external injury, and that most of these factors are immediately related to emotional reactions not only of the subject in pain but also of others to whom the subject has strong emotional attachments. Pain is closely related to empathy, a link that has been demonstrated not only in humans but also in experimental animals.

The concept of pain modulation strongly challenges the Cartesian notion that pain is only an alarm system—an injury pulls a cord and the pain bell rings in your brain. Modulation implies that the same kind of injury may pull the same cord several times with the same intensity and sometimes the bell may not ring at all, sometimes it may ring a little, and occasionally it may ring a lot, the final result depending on the emotional state of the person as well as on other factors at the time of each pull. The Cartesian model is very rigid and offers little opportunity for modulation, though it must be said that Descartes also recognized the influence of emotions and thoughts in sensory perception. After his famous description of the cord and the bell, he also wrote: "The same action that is agreeable to us when we are in good humor can often displease us when we are sad and sorrowful." This was a hint of recognition, however small, that emotions can modulate the perception of pain.

The limitations of the alarm-system model led to alternative proposals in which pain modulation took center stage. The best-known and by far the most influential of these is the *gate control theory of pain mechanisms* (*gate theory* for short), published by Ronald Melzack and Patrick Wall in 1965. The gate theory was a reaction to the failure of the Cartesian model to account for the variability of pain perception. Therefore, its focus was on pain modulation, and the specifics of the actual proposal centered on the interactions between those brain mechanisms that are ultimately responsible for the variability of a pain experience.

From a mechanistic point of view, the basic idea of pain modulation implies that the output can be different from the input at every stage in the transmission of pain signals through the brain, and therefore that the final pain experience is variable and dependent on the modulation of the message along the pain pathway rather than preset and determined by a rigid transmission chain. Modulation is the product of intrinsic systems within the brain that generate a final pain experience by taking into account the activities of other brain areas concerned with emotional reactions or cognitive factors. In addition, some basic components of the

individual, including sex, ethnicity, and age, also contribute to the overall modulation of pain.

The gate theory proposed that incoming activity in large afferent fibers, mostly from tactile sensors, can reduce the traffic in the fine afferent fibers that carry pain-related signals, and that this interaction occurs at the very first synaptic relay in the dorsal horn of the spinal cord. Nerve impulses in tactile fibers can close a gate in the spinal cord to the signals in pain fibers and hence reduce their traffic. These changes at the spinal-cord relay are also subject to further modulation by brain activity, and therefore the first synaptic stage in the spinal cord is a crossroads for pain modulation. The final output toward the brain and hence to the eventual perception of the pain experience would be not a rigid transmission of impulses (the Cartesian cord being pulled); rather, it would be a result of considerable modulation and interaction between incoming messages and brain activity.

The gate theory was based on two fundamentally different principles, one theoretical and the other mechanistic. The theoretical proposal was that pain is not the product of a rigid and preset brain mechanism but the result of interactions between incoming sensory signals and brain activity. Therefore, the pain produced by the same event can be variable, depending on external circumstances and the internal brain state. This theoretical principle is correct, and because it drew attention to modulation it is generally regarded as the gate theory's best contribution. But the other element of the gate theory was the proposal of a very detailed mechanism to account for pain modulation at the first synaptic relay of the spinal cord, and unfortunately the suggested machinery was shown to be wrong. Scientists who tested the mechanism proposed by the gate theory couldn't find supporting evidence for the circuitry, and this led them to dismiss the whole theory—a clear case of throwing the baby out with the bath water.

Yet the gate theory, by bringing pain modulation and pathological pain into the forefront of research, has been extremely constructive, triggering a great deal of very productive research on the brain mechanisms of pain modulation and of abnormal pain sensations. And this is, without a doubt, the greatest legacy of the theory. The English neurologist Peter Nathan, in an insightful review of the theory published in 1976, wrote the best compliment ever given to the gate theory: "Ideas need to be fruitful; they do not have to be right. And curiously enough, the two do not necessarily go together."

Stress and Pain

The wounded soldiers at Anzio, like those studied by Silas Weir Mitchell during the American Civil War, had extensive injuries but felt no pain. The same is true of the nurse (mentioned in an earlier chapter) who lost her arm in Turkey. All were under extreme stress at the time of their injuries, and our explanation is that stress eliminates pain. But feeling pain is also stressful, and therefore the relationship between stress and pain is not as simple or unidirectional as it would seem at first. Think, for instance, of watching another person in pain, specially a loved one. That could be at least as stressful as feeling your own pain. And we now know that some remarkable events take place in the brain of a person who sees other people feeling pain.

There are two different approaches to the pain of others. One is cognitive and rational, a mental process by which we assess and analyze the pain. Physicians and other members of the medical profession often use this method to deal with the suffering they witness every day. The other approach is empathy (that is, sharing the emotions and feelings of the other person), an affective state that can be as powerful as feeling one's own pain. Brain-imaging studies of people observing loved ones receive painful stimuli have shown that the same brain networks are activated in both the person in pain and the empathizer—particularly areas, such as the anterior insula and the anterior cingulate cortex, that are involved in the affective components and the unpleasantness of the pain experience. Watching a loved one in pain activates the same brain regions and triggers the same emotional reaction as if we were feeling the pain ourselves.

Interestingly, the amplitude of the brain activation caused by empathy is also modulated by rational, emotional, and external factors, but if the empathizer believes that the pain is real it is not related to whether the pain experienced by a loved one is real or feigned . The intensity of our brain reaction to the pain of another person depends on the emotional relationship between the two people, on the type of pain suffered, on our ability to understand their situation, on the perceived fairness or unfairness of the process, on our previous pain experiences, and on the sex of the empathizer (women having, in general, stronger empathic reactions than men).

Therefore, the emotional component of pain can color the entire experience of our own pain or of watching the pain of a loved one. Stressful

situations trigger powerful emotional reactions, which in turn influence the perception of pain. Under extreme stress, pain tends to be reduced or even to vanish altogether; however, the stress produced by constant pain, by a debilitating painful disease, or just by empathizing with the pain of others can generate the opposite effect: an increase in pain sensitivity.

Let us first consider *stress-induced analgesia*, the reduction in pain sensation caused by stress such as that experienced by soldiers during combat and by other people in similarly extreme situations. This phenomenon has been known for a long time, but only in the last few decades it has been possible to identify the areas of the brain involved in this kind of pain control and some of the underlying mechanisms. We have learned that our brains have developed a system of internal pain control that uses neurotransmitters with actions similar to those of morphine and other opiates.

Evidence for an endogenous brain mechanism of pain control was first obtained in the early 1970s. Scientists noticed, in experimental animals, that electrical stimulation of an area in the brain stem known as the *periaqueductal gray matter* produced an analgesia similar to that produced by a dose of morphine. Further studies showed that the effects of this stimulation were mediated by a descending pathway from the brain stem to the spinal cord that reduced the transmission of pain signals at this first synaptic relay. These observations led to the proposal that the brain had a powerful mechanism of pain inhibition that originated in the brain stem and acted via a descending pathway to cut off incoming impulses to the central nervous system at the level of the spinal cord. This network was labeled the *endogenous pain-control system.*

A few years later, there were two more breakthroughs. First, several groups of scientists in the United States and Europe found that morphine and other powerful opiates acted directly on the brain by binding to specific opioid receptors distributed through many brain areas, including the portion of the brain stem at the origin of the descending pain-control pathway. The second important observation was that the morphine antagonist naloxone was able to reverse the analgesia induced by electrical stimulation of the periaqueductal gray matter, thus giving a functional role for the opioid receptors of the endogenous pain-control system. This work led to the discovery of the brain's own opiate substances, the endogenous opioids, which included families of molecules and receptors (known popularly as *endorphins*) located in the brain and in other tissues. The interpretation of all these results is that the brain can stop the trans-

mission of the pain signals that arrive at the spinal cord by way of a descending pathway from the brain stem, and that this process involves the actions of opiate-like transmitters that are normally present in the regions of the brain that control pain.

In recent decades, a considerable amount of research work has shown that, as might have been expected, things aren't as simple as that interpretation suggests. There are indeed endogenous opioid transmitters in the brain, but their roles go far beyond that of pain control and include many other emotional and sensory outcomes. That most pain control happens at the spinal-cord relay by means of descending inhibitory pathways is also uncertain, as the opportunities for such modulation occur all along the central nervous system. Other neurotransmitters, and not only the endogenous opioids, have been shown to play important roles in pain modulation by the brain. But the basic idea of a powerful system within the brain capable of reducing or even stopping pain perception is still valid and has contributed a great deal to our understanding of stress-induced analgesia and related phenomena. That endogenous opioids are involved in this process is beyond doubt, but harnessing this knowledge into therapies for pain relief remains a challenge.

The stress caused by pain itself can also reduce pain perception. *Counter-irritation*, whereby restricted and controlled pain is induced by generating blisters, scratching the skin, applying irritant chemicals, or creating bruises and swellings by cupping, has been used therapeutically for centuries. The therapeutically controlled pains contribute to reducing the pain felt as a result of injury or disease. The rationale is the well-known principle that pain relieves pain, a belief beautifully summarized by the friendly advice given to Romeo that as "one fire burns out another's burning, one pain is lessened by another's anguish."

The mechanism thought to be responsible for the pain-relieving properties of pain itself is known as *diffuse noxious inhibitory controls* (DNIC). It was discovered in experimental animals when scientists observed that nociceptive neurons in the spinal cord were powerfully inhibited by painful stimuli applied anywhere else within the body; hence the qualifier *diffuse*. These observations were followed by findings that in human subjects a painful stimulus applied to any part of the body reduced the intensity of the pain felt from another region. The internal brain mechanisms involve connections between the spinal cord and the brain stem which function by releasing endogenous opioid transmitters.

The phenomenon of DNIC is a component of the protective aspects of pain perception as it focuses our attention on the more intense feelings

of pain in preference over less intense painful sensations. It also provides an explanation for counter-irritation therapies and even for procedures such as acupuncture. Patients suffering from fibromyalgia and from certain other functional pain disorders have a reduced expression of DNIC, and this has been interpreted as a dysfunction of the endogenous pain-control system and therefore a potential explanation for the enhanced pain felt by these patients. DNIC can be triggered not only by strong pain but also by stimuli just above the pain threshold, such as vigorous exercise or strong physical therapy. These activities produce an effect popularly called "endorphin rush"—a feeling of well-being attributed to the release of endorphins. Interestingly, feelings similar to those of an endorphin rush also occur during and after orgasm, at a time when there is also a substantial reduction in pain sensitivity that has been recorded experimentally. Yes, the pain sensitivity of humans while having sex has been measured in a laboratory.

The other side of the coin is that stress can also generate pain. The immediate reaction to an acutely stressful situation is pain reduction, but persistent stress leads to chronic pain. Stress-induced hyperalgesia is believed to be the cause of functional pain disorders such as irritable bowel syndrome, interstitial cystitis, and chronic pelvic pain. Models of these conditions have been reproduced in experimental animals after extended periods of stress or as a consequence of a stressful situation earlier in their lives.

The brain mechanism of stress-induced hyperalgesia is thought to be persistent activity within the networks that process pain-related signals in the central nervous system. This mechanism would be similar, but with the opposite sign, to the endogenous analgesia system; in this case the pathways between the brain stem and the spinal cord would activate one another and would maintain a high level of excitability in the form of a positive feedback loop. Such loops have been identified at several brain levels. Surprisingly, they often involve the same neurotransmitters that are active in the pain-reduction networks.

The relationship between stress and pain is not straightforward. It involves both pain reductions and pain enhancements, depending on the situation and on the duration of the stressors. We are beginning to understand the brain mechanisms that mediate the influence of an emotional state on the pain experience and the role of stress in triggering these mechanisms. But the final pain experience depends critically on our molecular constitution and on the individual differences between us. And much of this, or perhaps all of it, is genetic.

Pain and Genetics

Thousands of people undergo open-heart surgery every year, but only a minority develop severe chronic pain as a result of the operation. The same is true of less traumatic surgeries, including mastectomies and hernia operations. These operations damage the tissues and nerves at the points of incision, but only a small proportion of patients end up with persistent pain as a result of this damage. And who develops chronic pain is not related to the difficulties of the surgery, to the possible complications of the procedure, or even to the skill of the surgeon. It all depends on individual, presumably genetic, variations.

Something similar happens with the effects of analgesic drugs on individual patients. Some patients are very sensitive to them and need low doses to reduce or completely eliminate their pain. Other patients are not responsive at all, and either the analgesics fail to work or large doses must be administered to produce a relatively minor effect. Individual variations are problematic not only for the identification of who is likely to develop chronic pain but also for the assessment of the patients' response to analgesic treatment.

We tend to blame the genetic makeup of the individual for these variations, but when we look at the overall picture of a particular pain condition we also note that the socioeconomic backgrounds of the patients, their educational levels, their family situations, and even where they live are important factors in the generation of the pain disease. So is it genetics, or is it the environment? Nature or nurture?

The more we know about genetics, the more we realize that many aspects of our lives, including our susceptibility to suffer from certain diseases, are determined by our genetic composition. And we also think that the extent and intensity of our pain experiences and the likelihood that we may end up developing chronic pain are determined by our genetic background. This genetic determinism compromises one of our most beloved assets: our free will. Do our genes determine everything we will ever do or achieve? Can we modify what is already planned for us in our genetic material?

Current opinion on the relevance of genetics to pain perception is mixed. On the one hand, we have gathered an impressive array of data suggesting that the response to pain and the tendency to develop chronic pain are, to a large extent, genetically determined. On the other hand, we also believe, or perhaps just hope, that we can make changes in this genetically determined path by changing our behavior—for example, by

deliberately doing certain things to improve our health or by changing our diet or our lifestyle. Interestingly, we have also learned that these activities can, in turn, alter our genetic composition and improve the prospects of our offspring. Nature and nurture interact in such a way that we can still preserve the dream that we have free will.

The influence of genetics on pain perception is not only beyond doubt, it is also astonishing. For instance, a mutation that eliminates one of the molecules that regulate the movement of sodium across excitable cells—the one known as the *Na$_v$1.7 sodium channel*—results in complete insensitivity to pain. The lack of function of this one molecule results in a total loss of pain sensitivity. And mutations that generate an overactive Na$_v$1.7 sodium channel produce congenital diseases characterized by an increased pain sensitivity restricted to some parts of the body, hands, feet, or the perineal area. Other genes have been identified as responsible for painful diseases (including peripheral neuropathies and migraine) or for a predisposition to develop neuropathic pain after a herpes infection or as a consequence of diabetes. And the list of genetically determined pain conditions grows longer every day.

One set of observations about genetic influences on pain perception made the news a few years ago. People with red hair were found to have a different pain sensitivity and a different response to analgesics than people with brown, black, or blond hair. The initial report triggered a lot of research interest. Uniform results weren't obtained, but it is now thought that the same gene that determines the redness of a person's hair is also involved in the modulation of pain perception and the sensitivity of the person to analgesics and to anesthetics.

We are still far from understanding fully how genetics influences pain perception. Experimental studies try to identify these influences by looking at the behavior of genetically modified animals or by detecting which genes are active during a pain condition. But changing the genome of an animal inevitably produces compensatory changes that obscure the question under study, and some genetically modified animals develop so many abnormalities that either they can't survive or it is impossible to attribute their behavior to a single deficit.

Identifying which genes are responsible for the development of an experimentally induced pain condition isn't easy. Studies often show that hundreds of genes are active in the nervous system at the time pain develops, and it is hard to focus on just a few. Yet human studies tell us that a mutation affecting a single molecule can render people completely insensitive to pain. Advances are being made in pain genetics through

the use of experimental animals, but only when we show the relevance of individual genes to human pain we will be able to find a possible therapeutic approach to modify the genetic component of pain perception.

One possibility that it is being actively explored is that analgesic treatments should be tailored to an individual's genetic profile, a process known as *personalized medicine*. If we are able to identify the genetic factors that determine the pain response of each individual and its sensitivity to analgesics, then we can develop a specific treatment program for each patient. This applies not only to the actual pain experience of each person but also to the genetic influence on his or her ability to modulate the pain. We think that some forms of chronic pain develop as a result of dysfunctions of the individual's endogenous pain-control systems, which are also under the governance of his or her genetic constitution.

One of the most obvious genetic differences between individuals is their sex—that is, whether they are genetically male or female. As would be expected, there are considerable variations between the two sexes in their experiences of pain and in their emotional responses to it. And there are also variations in sensitivity to analgesic drugs and in the therapeutic effectiveness of analgesics.

Male and Female Pain

One of my colleagues maintains that someday analgesics will come in two colors: pink pills for women and blue pills for men. Indeed, there is a lot of truth in the observation that the experience of pain and the sensitivity to analgesic drugs differ significantly between males and females.

First, the nature and the location of pain originating from an organ not shared by the two sexes shows fundamental differences. Male-specific pain (testicular, prostatic, penile) is rare and is mostly associated with disease, but female-specific pain is an intrinsic and unavoidable component of a woman's life. Menstrual pain is a feature of the normal reproductive cycle, a monthly occurrence throughout the reproductive years. Childbirth is also a painful experience under normal circumstances, and even the initiation of sexual activity involves pain.

Then there is the quality of the pain. Contrary to popular belief, women have a lower pain threshold and a more intense affective response to pain than men. Women may be more used to feeling pain, but their

reaction to it is very emotional and their ratings of the unpleasantness of pain are always higher than those of men. And it is the emotional component of pain, more than the simple sensory experience, that makes it particularly unbearable. Pain in women has a very negative affective element that makes its experience very different from and more unpleasant than pain in men.

There are also differences in the prevalence of painful diseases. Migraine, fibromyalgia, irritable bowel syndrome, interstitial cystitis, and chronic pelvic pain are among the many diseases that are far more prevalent in women than in men. For some of these conditions, female prevalence approaches 80 percent of cases. And women are less sensitive to some analgesics than men.

What is the biological basis of these differences? A frequently explored option is the hormonal contingent of either sex. Males have testosterone, a sex hormone that is produced throughout a man's life (though the amount decreases with the years) and maintains the male sexual characteristics, including perhaps its reaction to pain. Females have estrogen and progesterone, whose production oscillates with the menstrual cycle and whose blood levels fluctuate in the course of a month. The female hormonal cycle causes changes of all kinds, from physical changes to mood variations. It is tempting to think that the variable pain response of women is linked to the menstrual cycle and therefore to changes in the levels of female hormones.

There have been many studies of pain sensitivity in women during the various phases of the menstrual cycle and many attempts to correlate the magnitude of pain perception with estrogen or progesterone levels at each time point. Unfortunately, there is little uniformity in the result of these studies, and we can't say for sure whether pain sensitivity is directly linked to these cyclic hormonal variations. Studies in experimental animals (such as rats and mice) that have shorter cycles have also been inconclusive. We aren't even certain from the available data whether estrogen reduces pain or exacerbates it. Nevertheless, clinical studies of pain conditions and diseases that are more prevalent in women have yielded some interesting data that support the idea of a direct involvement of sex hormones in the female response to pain.

Women suffering from fibromyalgia or from irritable bowel syndrome experience variations in the pain produced by their conditions throughout their menstrual cycle. The most frequent observation is that the pain is worst in the days just before menstruation, which makes the premenstrual period even more difficult than in healthy women. But the pain of

these diseases improves and is felt with reduced intensity and unpleasantness in the days immediately after menstruation.

A persuasive explanation for these observations is that it is the change in the levels of sex hormones that generates the variations of pain sensitivity, rather than the absolute levels of these hormones in the circulating blood. The sign of these changes is in favor of estrogen's having a helpful or protective role. When estrogen levels are rapidly decreasing, just before menstruation, is when the pain is felt at its worse. When the level of estrogen in the blood increases, just after menstruation, the pain lessens. This dynamic interpretation would also explain why it is difficult to correlate an absolute and static level of estrogen with a particular pain sensitivity; the problem seems to be that the hormonal changes are the cause of the variations in sensitivity to pain and, especially, in the emotional reaction to pain.

If absolute levels of estrogen were necessary to reduce pain sensitivity, it would follow that all postmenopausal women should develop pain-related diseases, as their levels of estrogen would be very low. It is true that some persistent pain conditions, including chronic pelvic pain, are frequent among postmenopausal women; however, many such women are pain free, and the same pain conditions can occur before menopause. Thus, it isn't possible to establish a direct parallel between estrogen levels and chronic pain. Yet female-related pain diseases, the level of estrogen or other sex hormones, and the presence of stress seem to be linked. Many diseases are worsened by added stress, and treatments aimed at reducing stress or improving the quality of life of the patients also produce beneficial pain-relieving effects. One such treatment is estrogen-replacement therapy, which not only improves the lives of postmenopausal women physically and psychologically but also reduces pain if there is an underlying functional pain condition.

What the pain-suppressing effects of stress documented at the Anzio beachhead and the beneficial actions of estrogen replacement have in common is that pain is a very variable sensation whose final experience depends on multiple internal and external factors, including genes, hormones, emotions, and stress. We are not far from the day when we will be able to make sense of the knowledge we are gathering about pain modulation and to use it effectively to design new methods of pain relief. Perhaps we will be able to modify how genes operate, or perhaps we will manage to harness the brain's response to stress. Or we may finally understand the differences between male and female pain and produce my colleague's blue and pink analgesic pills.

10 A Pain-Free World: Curing Pain

King Philip II of Spain, the ruler of one of the largest empires that the world has ever known, died on September 13, 1598, after a horrific agony that lasted nearly two months. During his reign he was king not only of Spain but also of Portugal, Sicily, Naples, and the Low Countries, and for a while even of England and Ireland. His overseas empire extended throughout the Americas, from California to Patagonia and also included territories in Africa and Asia. The Philippine Islands were not only part of his vast empire; they were also named after him. He was without doubt one of the most powerful men of his time.

He lived in a few small and austere rooms in a monastery attached to a huge basilica in the town of El Escorial, near Madrid . A champion of the Roman Catholic Church, he took it upon himself to rid the world of Protestants, heretics, and other such sinful creatures by waging religious wars, on which he squandered the vast treasures that arrived in Spain from the New World. If you visit the monastery in El Escorial, you will notice the harshness of King Philip's rooms, very small and modestly appointed yet embedded in a huge church lavishly decorated with silver and gold. His bedroom was tiny and windowless, decorated only with religious symbols. A small opening in one wall enabled him to see the altar of the basilica from his bed, to which he was confined toward the end of his life. There he died a horrible death, suffering for two months from unbelievable pain, caused mainly by gout but also by the ulcers and pustules that covered his body. The pain was so intense that he couldn't cover his body with a sheet or even leave the bed to relieve himself. There was a fetid and unbearable odor surrounding his body, and his aides couldn't approach him. A ghastly scene of pain that lasted for weeks until he finally died.

The point of this story is that King Philip's agony was unnecessary and avoidable. He was a powerful man, had access to the best physicians and

treatments of his time, and could have asked for a painless and speedy exit. His doctors were familiar with the medical properties of laudanum, a mixture of opium and alcohol that had long been known to be effective in relieving pain and to ease the transit to the other world. But Philip rejected any form of pain relief, believing, as a devout Catholic, that his agony was God's punishment for his sins and that enduring this pain would be necessary on his way to heaven. With no pain relief and no palliative care, he accepted with resignation and fortitude the pain that the Almighty had set aside for him.

Now let me tell you another story, equally true. This event happened only a few years ago, in 2008. The details were sent to me by a friend who runs a professional association dedicated to palliative care. Her email included a scan of a classified advertisement that had been published in a newspaper in the Colombian city of Cali. Among short notices of articles for sale and offers of personal services, an anonymous person had placed this ad: "Cancer kills us. Pain is killing me because for several days I cannot get morphine chlorhydrate 3% injectable anywhere. Please, Mr. Health Secretary, do not make us suffer anymore." The ad ended with a cell phone number.

What lessons can be drawn from these two stories? First, religious and other beliefs can get in the way of effective pain treatment, and when powerful or influential people hold these beliefs they can affect not only believers but also those under their authority. Second, we already have strong painkillers. The analgesic actions of opium have been known for centuries, and its active principle, morphine, was purified nearly 200 years ago. Third, many people today, as represented by the Cali advertiser, demand a more effective pain relief and no longer accept pain as an unavoidable component of disease. And there is a fourth and very important lesson: it is the responsibility of political leaders to ensure that the people they represent don't suffer needlessly, especially when they demand effective pain relief.

In this chapter I will discuss how pain can be relieved in our time while reflecting on the lessons of these two very different and very real stories.

Analgesics from Nature

The two most commonly used families of painkillers are both gifts of Mother Nature and have been known and used for a very long time. They are the opiates and the salicylates, represented by their leading products: morphine and acetylsalicylic acid (better known by its trade name,

aspirin). The opiates are strong painkillers, and their prescription is severely controlled because they are also drugs of abuse. Many of the salicylates, on the other hand, are widely available as over-the-counter medications, and all of them, including aspirin, have anti-inflammatory properties in addition to their analgesic activity.

Use of the latex of the opium poppy for medical or recreational purposes is nearly as old as the human race. The analgesic properties of this plant product have been known for centuries and have been part of the medical and social traditions of most cultures throughout time. The juice obtained from opium poppies contains several opiates, the most abundant of which is morphine, isolated and identified in the earlier years of the nineteenth century and commonly used as a painkiller. Many other opiates have been identified over the years, some of them natural products of the opium poppy (e.g. codeine), some of them semi-synthesized derivatives of morphine (e.g. heroin and oxycodone), and some of them fully synthesized artificially (e.g. methadone, fentanyl, and pethidine). The opiates are regarded as the "gold standard" of analgesia, and all new analgesics are measured by reference to the potency of morphine. Opiates act by binding to the molecular receptors that are present in neurons in many regions of the brain, including those concerned with the processing of pain-related signals. But because these receptors are widely distributed throughout the brain and in other tissues of the body, the opiates can also induce such undesirable side effects as euphoria, sleep, respiratory depression, nausea, vomiting, itch, and constipation.

Each opiate has its good points. Some are very fast acting and have short-lived effects; others have long-lasting effects and build up slowly in the organism. However, all of them have two unwelcome properties: addiction and tolerance. Physical addiction compels the user to keep taking the drug, and its withdrawal generates strong and unpleasant physical symptoms. Addiction to opiates is more frequent in people who take them for recreational use and can be avoided in carefully monitored patients who use them for pain relief, even those who take them for long periods of time. On the other hand, tolerance—that is, the reduction in effectiveness of the drug with repeated use and the need to increase the dose in order to obtain the same beneficial effects—is difficult to manage or avoid. The possibility of generating addiction and the potential for tolerance have made long-term use of opiates controversial. Few people would argue against their use in palliative care to ease the last days of a terminally ill patient, but their use as painkillers in people with long life expectancies or with non-life-threatening diseases is very much a topic

of debate, subject to the political, social, and religious beliefs of governments and individual citizens. Even so, many medical organizations have begun to campaign for better and wider use of opiates (particularly morphine) to treat all forms of severe pain, not only to reduce suffering but also as a cheap and easy way to manage pain if appropriate controls are in place.

Another undesirable consequence of long-term use of opiates is opiate-induced hyperalgesia, the opposite of pain relief. The mechanisms of this strange phenomenon aren't fully understood but are thought to involve processes similar to those that mediate sensitization of central-nervous-system neurons, including hyperactivity of the pathways that transmit pain-related information. Not everyone agrees that hyperalgesia is a frequent or even a real consequence of the long-term use of opiates, but the possibility remains that these pain-relieving drugs can also generate pain in the long term.

The other family of popular painkillers is the salicylates, a subset of a larger collection of substances with analgesic properties called *nonsteroidal anti-inflammatory drugs* (NSAIDs). The best-known member of the salicylates is acetylsalicylic acid (aspirin). The generic family name of the salicylates comes from the Latin word *salix*, which means "willow tree." The bark of that tree contains the active principle, salicylic acid. Extracts of willow bark have been used for centuries in many cultures, not only as analgesics but also to reduce fever and inflammation. The therapeutic constituents of willow bark were identified and isolated nearly 200 years ago and since then have become some of the most used medicines of all time, not only because of their analgesic and anti-inflammatory properties but also because they can reduce blood clotting and thus help to prevent strokes and heart attacks.

Aspirin and other members of the NSAID family (including ibuprofen and indomethacin) act at the site of inflammation, inhibiting the enzymes that produce and activate pro-inflammatory substances (the culprits in nociceptor sensitization and in the generation of the inflammatory pain). Unfortunately, inhibiting these enzymes also generates some adverse effects, among them gastric bleeding. Another drawback of NSAIDs is that most of them have the potential to trigger severe allergic reactions. To reduce these side effects, newer NSAIDs were developed; some of them turned out to increase cardiovascular risks and were withdrawn from the market. In any case, NSAIDs remain the first line of defense against many forms of pain, particularly pain that has a strong inflammatory component.

There are more natural products, besides opiates and salicylates, with strong analgesic properties. The psychoactive actions of the constituents of cannabis have been known for a long time, but only recently it has been found that the brain has endogenous receptors that bind with the active principles of this plant. These cannabinoid receptors are widely distributed in the peripheral and the central nervous system, including the regions that deal with pain processing, and synthetic cannabinoid products are now being studied for use as painkillers in the treatment of fibromyalgia, peripheral neuropathic pain, and other pain-producing conditions.

Another natural source of pain treatment is the chili pepper. As has already been noted, nociceptors in the skin, in muscles, and in internal organs have receptors for capsaicin, the pungent constituent of hot peppers. Repeated application of capsaicin desensitizes these sensors and reduces their activity. Capsaicin-containing patches and creams and synthetic antagonists of the capsaicin receptor have been developed for the purpose of easing the pain of conditions characterized by enhanced nociceptor activity, including arthritis and some forms of neuropathic pain.

It is enlightening to know that the human brain has developed pain-reducing mechanisms based on the actions of the molecular components of certain plants. Pain originally appeared as a defense reaction to protect us against a hostile environment, and much of this hostility comes from the irritants and toxics produced by animals and plants. In the process of dealing with these threats, we have developed mechanisms to decrease pain sensitivity that are also based on using products from our environment. This closes an interesting adaptive loop in which the external threats and the brain mechanisms that deal with them make use of the same molecular constituents.

We have also been smart enough to turn environmental hostility to our advantage. There is a family of sea snails, known as cone snails, that kill their prey by projecting a harpoon-like appendage and injecting toxins. These conotoxins contain substances that block the ionic channels of the cells of the prey, making the ionic channels unexcitable and thus paralyzing and killing the victim. These properties of conotoxins have been applied to develop a synthetic derivative, called ziconotide, that is now used as an effective painkiller in cases of severe chronic pain arising from hyperexcitability of the central nervous system. Ziconotide is injected directly into the cerebrospinal fluid of the patient, where it reduces the excitability of the nervous system, thus decreasing the

sensitivity to pain. The process of administration of this therapy is cumbersome, and the cost is very high, but here is a clever example of using toxins developed by nature to improve our methods of pain relief.

Analgesics or Anti-Hyperalgesics?

A common element of the therapeutic properties of opiates and salicylates is that they are both analgesics—that is, they reduce pain sensitivity. The opiates act at a high brain level, breaking the link between pain perception and the unpleasant emotional reaction that normally accompanies pain so that under the influence of opiates pain is less unpleasant. The salicylates, on the other hand, reduce inflammatory reactions as well as the sensitivity of peripheral nociceptors, and this causes a general decrease in pain sensitivity. The problem with both groups of drugs is that they reduce all forms of pain, both the good and the bad, and by doing so they make us vulnerable to the hostility of the environment because our pain alarm bell is no longer in good working order. Eliminating all pain is fine if you don't have to drive a car, operate machinery, or just go about your normal life, but for most pain conditions it would be much more helpful to reduce or remove the bad pain—the increased pain sensitivity—while leaving the ability to feel normal protective pain intact.

These considerations have moved the therapeutic emphasis of pain treatment from analgesia (elimination of pain sensitivity) to anti-hyperalgesia (reduction of the enhanced pain sensitivity caused by injury or disease). Today we want medications with fewer side effects; more important, we want painkillers that don't impair our capacity to feel normal pain and that maintain its protective aspect. This is particularly important in chronic pain, and especially in neuropathic pain, where the underlying disease lasts for a very long time and the treatments are likely to be long term. We should not weaken the protective aspect of pain in our patients for the rest of their lives.

The treatment of neuropathic pain is a good example of the problems associated with the long-term use of conventional painkillers. The received knowledge among medical professionals is that opiates don't work, or don't work very well, in neuropathic pain conditions. Larger doses are needed to generate effective pain relief, and larger doses produce many unwanted side effects. Opiates are not widely used to treat neuropathic pain. Nonsteroidal anti-inflammatory drugs (NSAIDs) are also ineffective against neuropathic pain, even that caused or accompa-

nied by an inflammatory process. It seems that when the brain mechanism that generates a pain experience breaks down, a novel set of therapeutic approaches must be used to mend the faulty machine. And here is where anti-hyperalgesics can be very useful.

The most popular first line of defense against neuropathic pain is the use of antidepressant drugs, including the classic amitryptiline and the more modern dulaxetine. These medications interfere with the normal function of some important brain transmitters—particularly norepinephrine and serotonin, each of which is known to play an important role in the triggering of the endogenous pain-control system Although many of the drugs in this category were originally developed for use as antidepressants, most have analgesic and anti-hyperalgesic effects and are the medications of choice for treating chronic pain, particularly chronic pain that is of neuropathic origin. Their pain-relieving actions are linked to their mood-changing effects and to general improvement in the quality of life of the patient. They are not painkillers in a classical sense, but they help to reduce the unpleasantness and the negative emotional component of neuropathic pain. Occasionally, drugs of this type are used in combination with mild opiates to treat chronic pain.

The proposal that hyperalgesia is a consequence of increased excitability of the neurons in the central nervous system that transmit injury-related information has led to the idea that chronic pain may be produced by a mechanism similar to the one that triggers epileptic attacks. In both cases there would be uncontrolled and widespread excitation of brain neurons, resulting in convulsions in the case of epilepsy and increased pain sensitivity when the hyperexcitability affects areas of the central nervous system that mediate the perception of a pain experience. This is why some drugs developed originally as anticonvulsants or to reduce neuronal excitability have also proved effective in managing chronic pain. This category includes the drugs gabapentin and pregabalin, widely used to treat many neuropathic pain conditions and to treat fibromyalgia and other functional pain states.

A special case in the development of medications for the treatment of chronic pain is that of migraine. This is still a mysterious condition. Its mechanisms aren't fully understood, and until recently, there were no very effective treatments for it. However, the triptans—a new class of drugs developed in the last few decades—have proved highly beneficial in stopping or reducing migraine attacks. The triptans are successful products of research targeted at a specific mechanism, in this case the decrease in the production of a neuropeptide that is known to play a role

in a migraine attack. Triptans don't cure migraine but can stop an attack quickly; if taken at the right time, they can even prevent an attack.

Trying to reduce the enhanced excitability of the nervous system in a hyperalgesic state has also led to using more direct ways of administering drugs. In some cases, direct application of patches containing local anesthetics (such as lidocaine) to a hyperalgesic area manages to reduce the hyperactivity of the nociceptors and reduce incoming painful signals to the brain. Another popular approach is to inject the excitability-reducing drug directly in the cerebrospinal fluid or in the space surrounding the spinal cord (epidural injections), hoping to interfere with the transmission of pain signals through the first synaptic relay or to stimulate the descending pain-control pathways. Spinal injections (either direct or by means of implanted catheters and continuous delivery with pumps) is also a popular treatment for intense pain that doesn't respond to oral medications. The catheters are expensive and difficult to install and maintain, but they offer a useful alternative based on direct action of the drugs on the hyperactive area of the central nervous system.

Without losing sight of the excellent pain-relieving properties of opiates and nonsteroidal anti-inflammatories, we have moved toward the use of drugs that control the increased excitability of the nervous system, which we believe is the cause of chronic pain. It is hoped that in the near future we will be able to reduce hyperalgesia while maintaining normal pain sensitivity and thus to control chronic pain without adversely affecting pain's usefulness as an alarm signal.

Pain Relief without Drugs

The ancient Greeks recommended standing on an electric fish as a method of relieving pain. Trepanation (removal of circular sections of bone from the skull) and other crude surgical procedures were once used for a variety of reasons including pain relief. Acupuncture, massage, yoga, and meditation have also been used to treat pain. There is indeed a long list of non-pharmacological techniques for the treatment of pain.

Surgical procedures aimed at pain relief range from nerve blocks to sections of brain pathways to frontal lobotomy. Surgeons, ancient and modern, are not the most cautious people when it comes to cutting up the nervous system, and the list of operations that have been carried out in various attempts to control pain is quite long. The most radical of the surgeries are those that involve destruction of very important areas of the brain, including the pituitary gland, the thalamus, and the hypothala-

mus, and those that aim to interrupt pain pathways within the central nervous system at the spinal, the brain-stem, or the cerebral level. Virtually all such operations are performed as a last resort in patients with severe pain that doesn't respond to pharmacological treatment and with very short life expectancy. The effectiveness of these operations is controversial, especially when performed in patients with longer life expectancy, and their use is restricted to very specific cases when the end of life is very close, the pain is excruciating, and all other forms of treatment have failed.

Less radical surgeries aimed at the peripheral nervous system involve nerve blocks (permanent or temporary) and removal of neuromas from severed nerves. The rationale for these procedures is that the pain is coming from hyperexcitable peripheral nerves (normal or damaged), and that blocking the traffic of impulses in these nerves or removing the sources of abnormal activity will reduce the enhanced excitability that these impulses cause when they arrive in the central nervous system. Nerves can be blocked temporarily with local anesthetics and more permanently with alcohol or by applying intense cold or radio-frequency signals. Mixed surgical and pharmacological procedures involve injecting anti-inflammatory drugs or even opiates or other analgesics close to a peripheral nerve. The evidence for the efficacy of these procedures is controversial. Some doctors claim that the ritual of the treatments, which involve imposing equipment, operating rooms, and associated paraphernalia, can induce improvements in the patients' conditions through suggestion rather by a scientifically identifiable mechanism.

Another group of non-pharmacological techniques involve the use of electrical currents. The most popular method, *transcutaneous electrical nerve stimulation* (TENS), was developed as a corollary of the gate control theory. According to that theory, impulses in the large afferent fibers that transmit touch-related signals close a gate in the spinal dorsal horn to the traffic of impulses in pain nerve fibers. Therefore, artificial activation of tactile nerve fibers in peripheral nerves by electrical stimulation will block incoming messages in pain fibers and thus reduce pain. The efficacy of these stimulators in relieving pain hasn't been fully demonstrated, as they seem to work better when the intensity of the electrical current is high enough to activate pain fibers and therefore more related to a process of counter-irritation than to the postulates of the gate theory. Nevertheless, alternatives to TENS using more permanent stimulators, with electrodes implanted in the spinal cord and aimed at activating tactile fibers on their way toward the brain, are still popular, having

shown a certain degree of effectiveness against chronic pain such as that of angina.

Deep brain stimulation by means of electrodes implanted in regions of the brain known to be involved in the modulation of pain has also been used for pain relief, as have similar procedures that activate the motor cortex and other non-sensory regions. The efficacy of these methods has been inconsistent, and the results have ranged from excellent pain relief to no relief at all. We still know very little about the workings of all these brain regions, and to stimulate them in a relatively crude way with electrical currents may not be the best way to engage the endogenous pain-control systems of the brain. The procedures are costly and therefore their use is not widespread.

An interesting approach to the treatment of phantom-limb pain involves mirrors and virtual reality. The rationale is that the patient that suffers from phantom-limb pain often feels the missing limb as being forced into an awkward position or permanently clinched or twisted. Providing the patient with visual images suggesting that the missing limb is in a normal and relaxed position helps to reset the body image that is causing the pain. This can be done with mirrors: the patients see an image of their good limb reflected on a mirror that is located where the missing limb once was. Therefore the patients can move and observe what they think is their missing limb when they move their good limb. Other approaches use virtual reality to make the patient believe that the missing limb is still there and that it can be moved normally and placed in a relaxed and comfortable position. The effectiveness of these techniques is still under evaluation, but the initial reports are promising and offer an exciting avenue for non-pharmacological treatment of this terrible form of neuropathic pain.

Discussing alternative (or complementary, as they are now called) therapies for pain relief is always difficult. Opinions are strong, either way, and evidence of effectiveness is far from conclusive. Acupuncture and other complementary techniques have been around for hundreds of years but aren't based on mechanisms that can be identified and tested by the scientific method. Relaxation, yoga, and therapeutic massage improve the quality of life, and that may be sufficient to reduce pain's unpleasantness and intensity. It we take a non-committal point of view, we can say that any procedure that doesn't harm the patient must be either good or neutral and therefore there should be no obstacles to trying these innocuous techniques. If a patient's pain is reduced by a complementary technique and no harm is done, then its use is justified.

An inquiring mind will still wonder why these methods work and how they bring forward an element of our brain function that relieves pain. And studying why and how these procedures work may also help to unravel some of the brain's more enigmatic functions.

Perhaps the most spectacular method of non-pharmacological pain relief involves the placebo response: a positive reaction of the body to a pretend medical procedure. For example, a patient is given pills that don't contain any active principle but with a strong suggestion that they will reduce pain—and they do. Similarly, using a stimulator with no batteries or making injections with complicated machinery but without any drug can reduce pain when the patient is told that it is an effective method of pain relief. Causing a reduction in pain sensitivity by the suggestion of a faked therapeutic intervention is a very impressive phenomenon that can be induced in a large proportion of the population. Estimates of how many normal individuals are susceptible to placebo responses range from 10 percent to 50 percent.

The placebo response is real and can be induced either by expectation of a positive outcome ("Taking this pill will ease my pain") or by conditioning of a certain situation ("The doctor is always right and wants to help me"). Brain-imaging studies have demonstrated that people responding to a placebo show reductions of brain activity in the regions normally activated by a painful event; therefore, the placebo response is part of the normal processing of pain and of the endogenous pain-control system of the brain. Studies have also shown that the placebo response involves the actions of neurotransmitters, such as dopamine or serotonin, that mediate reward reactions, and perhaps the activation of endogenous opioid receptors. Even the color of a placebo pill contributes to its expected action; people expect a stimulant if the pill is red and a relaxant if it is a pastel color. We still know little about how the placebo response works, and we haven't yet managed to harness its therapeutic potential for pain relief.

A Pain-Free World?

A question that I often ask my students when we discuss pain mechanisms is "What is the strongest pain that you have ever felt?" This question is always followed by a long period of silence, much thinking and searching, and, if we are lucky, by a reply like "Well . . . I once twisted my ankle while skiing and it hurt a lot or I had a really bad headache one day after I got very drunk." A more common reply is "I can't really

recall having felt much pain in my whole life." The obvious conclusion is that nowadays healthy young people living in a developed country are exposed to very little pain. But on one occasion something unusual happened. One of my students said, calmly and without any sign of concern, that the most intense pain that he had ever felt had come when a dentist removed two of his teeth. The other students, rather alarmed, asked about the circumstances of such intervention. Was it an emergency? An accident? The student who had made the statement couldn't understand why they were asking such questions. After a while, it became clear that the dentist had extracted the two teeth without any anesthesia or analgesia, and that the young man regarded that as normal. He was from a poor and underdeveloped country. To the horror of his classmates, he proceeded to tell them in some detail how dental procedures and other such surgical interventions are normally carried out in his country without any form of pain control or relief.

What this real story tells us is that how much pain we are prepared to tolerate depends critically on our previous pain experiences and on our expectations. Today thinking about having a tooth pulled without anesthesia makes us cringe, but not long ago that was a normal event not only in the remote parts of the world where it is still commonplace but everywhere. Local and general anesthesia are relatively recent developments. Only 100 years ago, James Mackenzie, a Scottish surgeon, published a book describing the pain experiences of people undergoing abdominal surgery. Mackenzie was able to obtain this information by direct report from his patients, on whom he was operating on without any anesthetic, local or general. To us having one's appendix removed without anesthetics is unimaginable, yet it was a common occurrence not very long ago.

As we improve our pain treatments and develop new and better analgesic procedures, we get caught in a vicious circle that makes a pain-free world an impossible goal. Society demands more and better analgesia, which leads to increased availability of pain-relief procedures, which in turn reduces the amount of pain around us and increases our expectations of a pain-free life. This produces a lower pain tolerance, and therefore an increased demand for more analgesia, a further reduction in the amount of pain around us, even lower pain tolerance, and so on. The final goal—no pain—gets progressively closer but is never reached.

We are moving in the direction of greater availability of pain-relief procedures, and therefore in the direction of reduced exposure to pain. We have to accept that there will always be a certain amount of pain

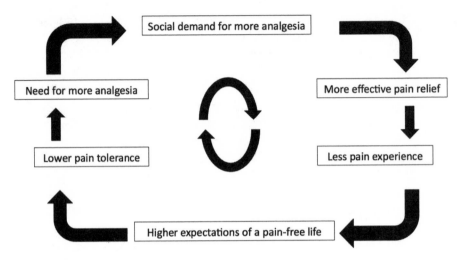

Figure 10.1
The vicious circle of pain relief.

around us, but we strive to decrease its effects on our lives and to diminish its unpleasantness. And in our journey toward a less painful existence we have to deal with three important obstacles: social, administrative, and scientific.

The first obstacle is our own society. I have already noted that modern society is changing its appreciation of what pain means to an individual. From thinking that pain is a test of character that must be endured with fortitude, society is moving toward thinking that there is no reason to suffer pain and that it is perfectly rational to get rid of it. Yet a large segment of the population is still influenced by religious and moral attitudes that regard pain not only as inevitable but also as a kind of mystic accomplishment. As the saying goes, "no pain, no gain." Changing this social perception requires strong and credible arguments to demonstrate how chronic pain ruins the lives of the sufferers, both physically and psychologically, and the lives of people close to them.

The second obstacle is administrative. We have powerful and effective pain treatments, but because of economic, political, or organizational difficulties they don't reach everyone in the world. There is no reason why teeth should still be extracted without any analgesia and anesthesia anywhere. Post-operative pain, the most common kind of acute pain, is easily treated and managed in a hospital if the resources, the organization, and the will are in place. Cancer pain can be effectively controlled so that people don't have to die in agony. This is the job of politicians

and administrators, health-care policy makers, and those who run hospitals and clinics. The means are there, and they aren't expensive. All that is needed is political will and organization.

An associated problem, more economic than administrative, has to do with the role of the pharmaceutical industry in the development of analgesic therapies. Because of the great expense of developing new medications, pharmaceutical companies are interested more in developing drugs that can generate substantial profits than in developing cheap and commercially uninteresting products. As a consequence, the industry is more interested in selling medicines in the developed countries, where profits are substantial, than in supplying them to poorer countries at low prices.

The relationship between the developed and the developing worlds in regard to the availability and distribution of analgesics is complex. A case in point is the availability of opiates, the most effective painkillers, whose use has been promoted very successfully in many developed countries. This has produced a substantial reduction of pain in these countries, but it also has led to unwanted effects associated with the long-term use of opiates and to addiction and abuse. And that has generated a backlash in developed countries, where strong warnings are heard about the dangers of making these drugs too easily available, and a knock-on effect in the developing world, where, owing to deficiencies in control and enforcement, opiates have become almost unavailable. The regulating authorities should be persuaded that there are clear indications for the proper use of opiates and that they should be available worldwide, under the correct medical management, to reduce pain.

The third obstacle is scientific, generated by the difficulties of developing new analgesics that target pain mechanisms (particularly those of persistent and chronic pain) and have few or no side effects. The traditional method has been to study pain (or, better, the responses of the nervous system to injury) in experimental animals and then translate these findings to the human pain experience. Much has been gained by this approach, but there have also been some spectacular fiascos in which new drugs developed on the basis of scientific data have failed to produce any analgesic effects in human patients. These failures have been blamed on the complexity of the human pain experience (which is very difficult to reproduce in an experimental animal) and on the fact that the final perception of human pain depends on a multitude of factors and not only on those that we share with other animal species.

How can something as elusive as pain—a complex experience that can only be measured by the verbal reports of patients—be studied

scientifically? This is without doubt the greatest question that pain scientists face today. It will not be answered until we develop objective methods for measuring pain and manage to understand the relationship between the cellular processes the central nervous system uses to process injury and the perception of the pain experience.

We now have very effective therapies that alleviate acute pain, postoperative pain, and the pain caused by injury. Making these treatments available throughout the world will require political will, organization, and some money. The therapies aren't expensive, and the task is achievable if we really want to reduce acute pain. We can also deal effectively with pain at the end of life. We can help to make the last weeks or days of a patient's life bearable and dignified. For this we need social acceptance and support and a new way of thinking of pain as an unwanted foe. We can also control some forms of chronic and persistent pain, although there is a large group of pain diseases against which much progress still needs to be made. The strong drugs we already have to control pain can't be used for long periods of time without harm and side effects. We need to develop better and safer therapies for the treatment of chronic pain.

What we do know is that no one should die the horrible death of King Philip, and that people such as the advertiser in Cali deserve to get the pain medications that will make their lives bearable. We may never achieve a pain-free world, but we must try.

Epilogue

We began our journey of inquiry into the mechanisms and meaning of pain with words of comfort from a loving mother to her young child in pain: "Big boys don't cry." These words told the little boy that pain is inevitable and that he would have to learn to accept it with resignation and courage. During our journey we asked many questions about the brain mechanisms that generate pain experiences and emotions, how these feelings are modified by external and internal factors, how can we ease and relieve pain, and what the experience of pain means to us as individuals and to society as a whole. What have we learned?

1. Pain is much more than a simple sensory experience. We describe it as a multi-dimensional phenomenon. It is physical, emotional, and rational, and it influences our life in many different ways. The experience of pain depends more on the background of a specific situation than on the magnitude of an underlying injury. We are likely to gain a full understanding of the neurological mechanisms that mediate these complex experiences soon, but we will always have to take into account all the other factors that condition the pain experience.

2. There are many different pains, and many different pain mechanisms. Nociceptive, inflammatory, and neuropathic pains are the big categories into which we classify pain, but we must make further distinctions and sub-classifications to accommodate all the various forms of normal and abnormal pain. Some brain mechanisms mediate more than one kind of pain, but others are very specific to individual kinds of pain. We are beginning to explore the more complex forms of pain experimentally, and we have found that it isn't easy to reproduce a human pain experience in an experimental setting. We have learned much from laboratory work, but we still need more clinical data from patients and more data from experimental studies of human subjects. It is imperative to maintain

an active path between the laboratory and the clinic so that the most distinctive features of human pain can be revealed through studies of the human brain.

3. We have learned a great deal over the years about the cellular and molecular processes that are triggered by injuries, by nerve lesions, and by inflammatory reactions. The contribution of laboratory scientists to the understanding of the neural mechanisms of injury has been, and still is, immense. Unfortunately, most experimental studies deal only with nociception (the brain's processing of injury-related information). How these mechanisms and processes generate the actual perception of the human pain experience is still unknown. We can record the electrical activities of neurons and their metabolic reactions, measure their chemical contents and the transmitters they release, and study their connectivity and their dynamic responses to sustained injury, but we still need to close the gap between highly reduced laboratory data and the complexity of a human pain experience. Succeeding in this task will be a giant step toward understanding the neural mechanisms of pain.

4. What pain means to each of us is critically dependent on our personal and collective history and on our religious, spiritual, and political beliefs. Modern society imposes fewer moral precepts and offers a greater freedom of individual values than traditional society. Our attitude toward pain has become less collective and more personal; you may wish to take a resigned attitude toward your pain, but I don't have to do the same. This new moral position based on personal choices offers a good opportunity for moving away from the traditional view that pain is inevitable and that we must accept it and learn to live with it.

5. Pain treatment should be considered a fundamental human right, and we should strive to persuade governments and health authorities that they should implement measures to reduce pain and suffering. Because we value human life, we want to enjoy it and improve its quality. There have been important advances in the social acceptance of pain relief aimed at easing the end of our lives and eliminating painful agonies. We have more and more powerful means of controlling pain that can be used safely at relatively low cost. The social attitude toward pain has shifted radically away from suffering in silence.

6. We will always need a pain bell at the end of the alarm cord to help us survive in a hostile environment. We know that the pain that protects us from injury and keeps us out of harm is good for us. But we are striving to eliminate the pain of disease, abnormal pain that is of no use to

us, and the persistent and chronic pain that ruins many lives. Unfortunately, the more pain we remove from the world, the less tolerance we have for the pain that remains, and that creates a vicious circle. We are constantly moving the goalposts of effective analgesia by reducing our tolerance of pain and making pain relief more and more difficult. It is possible that we will always have to live with a certain amount of pain, but the amount of pain we endure today is only a fraction of what our ancestors had to suffer in the recent past. Thus, we are moving in the right direction.

7. Seventy years ago Thomas Lewis told us that "pain is known to us by experience and described by illustration." That is true but unhelpful. Today we are getting close to being able to measure accurately the amount of a patient's pain and able to follow the success or failure of a treatment with objective tools. Brain imaging and associated techniques have revealed new opportunities for more precise assessment of pain. At about the same time that Lewis wrote these elegant but not very helpful words, Charles Sherrington expressed frustration by writing that pain "remains a biological enigma, a mere curse." Yet since then we have learned a great deal about the mechanisms the brain uses to detect injury, and we are rapidly approaching the possibility of developing personalized treatments that will deal not only with the sensory aspects of pain but also with its emotional components and with the genetic variations of each individual patient. Today we are more optimistic, pain is less of an enigma, and we are fighting it effectively.

We now approach the study and treatment of pain from a new and more helpful perspective. We believe that human suffering is unnecessary and avoidable, and that we must treat pain as a multi-dimensional disease and not just as a symptom. The mother in the playground should tell her injured son that crying when it hurts is perfectly natural and that, by the way, she has a cream that will heal his wound and take his pain away. And then our little boy, his mother, and all of us will be much happier and a great deal wiser.

Glossary

Allodynia Pain produced by stimuli that don't normally cause pain, among them touch and cold. Allodynia can be a normal process, as when lightly touching an injury site produces pain. But it can also be a symptom of disease. Some patients feel pain when uninjured parts of their bodies are touched or when they are exposed to small changes in temperature.

Endogenous opioids Substances, produced naturally by the brain and by other tissues — that modulate pain sensitivity. Their collective name indicates their similarity to the opiates (morphine, codeine, heroin) produced from plants such as the opium poppy, which bind to the same molecular receptors in the brain that are the targets of the endogenous opioids. They also fulfill other functions.

Functional pain Pain in the absence of an apparent cause (in contrast with *organic* pain, for which definite causes always can be found). Chronic pain states in which this occurs include those of irritable bowel syndrome, interstitial cystitis, and fibromyalgia.

Hyperalgesia An increase in pain sensitivity such that normally painful stimuli feel even more painful. An expression of enhanced pain sensitivity, it can be a normal consequence of an injury or a symptom of disease. When hyperalgesia occurs in an injured area, it is called *primary* hyperalgesia. When it develops in areas adjacent to, distant from, or remote from an injured area, or in the absence of injury, it is called *secondary* hyperalgesia.

Inflammatory pain Pain produced as a consequence of a peripheral inflammation, either acute or chronic. A normal kind of pain, associated with the healing of wounds, it can also become persistent, chronic, and pathologic.

Neuropathic pain Pain that arises as a consequence of a lesion or disease of the nervous system. It is always abnormal and is always due to malfunctioning of the nervous system, particularly of the somatosensory system (the part of the nervous system that deals with sensory signals from the body). If the lesion is restricted to peripheral nerves, the pain is called *peripheral* neuropathic pain. If the lesion is located in the central nervous system, it is called *central* neuropathic pain.

Nociception The process by which the nervous system detects and transmit injury-related information. It doesn't imply conscious perception of pain; it merely qualifies the neural process of detecting and processing an injury. Nociception describes the response of individual neurons or of a network of neurons to a painful stimulus, not the perception of the stimulus as painful.

Nociceptive pain Pain produced by the normal activation of nociceptors, either by an injury or by a potentially damaging stimulus. It is the normal response of the organism to an injury, and an alarm signal that warns of potential or actual harm.

Nociceptor-specific neurons One of the two types of neurons in the central nervous system that receive and transmit injury-related signals. Normally nociceptor-specific neurons are activated only by nociceptors and therefore by painful or potentially painful stimuli. During persistent pain states, however, they can also be activated by less intense

stimuli. Though distributed throughout the central nervous system, from the spinal cord to the brain cortex, they are less numerous than wide-dynamic range neurons.

Nociceptors   Sensors, distributed throughout the tissues of the body, that detect injury and transmit information about it to the central nervous system. Nociceptors encode chemical, mechanical, and thermal energy, but only within the range that is felt as painful. They are not specific for a single form of energy. Their adequate stimuli are those that are painful or potentially painful. Some nociceptors can be activated only by intense stimuli and become more excitable after an injury or after inflammation; these are called *silent* nociceptors.

Noxious stimulus   A stimulus that is damaging or potentially damaging. Most stimuli are defined by their type of energy (for instance, mechanical, thermal, or chemical). However a noxious stimulus is qualified by its capacity to produce an injury, regardless of the form of energy. Noxious stimuli are also called *nocuous*.

Pain   The International Association for the Study of Pain defines pain as an unpleasant sensory and emotional experience associated with actual or potential tissue damage, or described in terms of such damage. Pain is a multi-dimensional experience, sensory and emotional, always unpleasant, and associated (but not necessarily causally) with injury. When pain appears in the absence of injury, it is still described by the sufferer as if produced by injury.

Pattern theory of pain   A theoretical interpretation that proposes that pain is a result of the pattern of activation of peripheral sensors and central-nervous-system neurons and not of a chain of specific pain-related neurons. The emphasis of the pattern theory is on how brain neurons are activated by pain-producing stimuli rather than on what specific neurons are activated.

Phantom-limb pain   Pain felt in a limb that no longer exists.

Placebo response   A therapeutic effect achieved by the administration of a fake treatment. In the case of pain, placebo responses are reductions of pain sensation caused by procedures that don't contain active principles. Placebo responses can be achieved by suggestion, expectation, or conditioning.

Sensitization   A general term used in many scientific fields to qualify any process of enhanced activity whereby a system becomes more active and excitable. In pain research, it is used to describe the enhanced output of a nociceptive neuron after a period of intense stimulation. It is believed that sensitization underlies the increased pain sensitivity that appears in persistent and chronic pain states. Sensitization that occurs in peripheral nociceptors is called *peripheral sensitization*. Sensitization detected in neurons of the central nervous system is called *central sensitization*.

Specificity theory of pain   A theoretical interpretation of the mechanisms of pain that proposes that pain is a result of the orderly activation of a chain of neurons all of which are concerned with detecting and transmitting pain-related information. The emphasis of the specificity theory is on the type of neuron activated by a painful stimulus and on the existence of dedicated lines and networks within the brain that process injury-related signals.

Visceral pain   Pain caused by injury, disease, or inflammation of an internal organ. Caused only by certain stimuli (among them mechanical distension and ischemia), it can be evoked from only some of the internal organs. Many forms of visceral pain are normal defense reactions, but some diseases, including cancer, can also cause visceral pain.

Visual Analog Scale   A standard instrument for measuring pain in humans: a straight line, 10 centimeters long, with the words NO PAIN at one extreme (numbered 0) and WORST PAIN IMAGINABLE at the other (numbered 10). The subject rates his or her pain by making a mark at the appropriate point on the scale.

Wide-dynamic-range neurons   Neurons in the central nervous system that are activated by a variety of stimuli (both innocuous ones and noxious ones) and encode a wide range of stimulus intensities (some non-painful, some painful). They are the most numerous kind of nociceptive neurons in the central nervous system. Because they receive inputs from a large number of sources, they are also referred to as *convergent neurons*.

Index

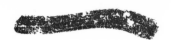